Calculating

Drug Doses Safely

A HANDBOOK FOR NURSES
AND MIDWIVES

This book should be returned by the last date stamped
above. You may renew the loan for a further period
if the book is not required by another reader.

For Elsevier:

Senior Commissioning Editor: Ninette Premdas
Project Development Manager: Mairi McCubbin
Project Manager: David Fleming
Designer: Judith Wright
Illustrations Manager: Bruce Hogarth

Calculating
Drug Doses Safely

A HANDBOOK FOR NURSES AND MIDWIVES

Professor George Downie MSc FRPharmS

Director of Pharmacy and Medicines Management, NHS Grampian, Aberdeen, UK

Jean Mackenzie BA(Open) RGN SCM DipN(Lond) RCT RNT

Formerly lecturer, School of Nursing and Midwifery, The Robert Gordon University, Aberdeen, Scotland, UK

Arthur Williams OBE FRPharmS

Formerly Chief Administrative Pharmaceutical Officer, Grampian, Orkney, Shetland and Tayside Health Boards, Scotland, UK

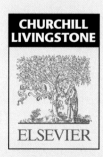

CHURCHILL LIVINGSTONE

ELSEVIER

EDINBURGH LONDON NEW YORK OXFORD PHILADELPHIA ST LOUIS SYDNEY TORONTO 2006

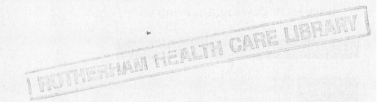

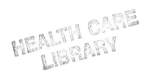

ELSEVIER | CHURCHILL LIVINGSTONE

An imprint of Elsevier Limited

© 2006, Elsevier Limited. All rights reserved.

First published 2006

ISBN 0443074607

British Library Cataloguing in Publication Data
A catalogue record for this book is available from the British Library

Library of Congress Cataloging in Publication Data
A catalog record for this book is available from the Library of Congress

Notice
Knowledge and best practice in this field are constantly changing. As new research and experience broaden our knowledge, changes in practice, treatment and drug therapy may become necessary or appropriate. Readers are advised to check the most current information provided (i) on procedures featured or (ii) by the manufacturer of each product to be administered, to verify the recommended dose or formula, the method and duration of administration, and contraindications. It is the responsibility of the practitioner, relying on their own experience and knowledge of the patient, to make diagnoses, to determine dosages and the best treatment for each individual patient, and to take all appropriate safety precautions. To the fullest extent of the law, neither the Publisher nor the authors assume any liability for any injury and/or damage to persons or property arising out of or related to any use of the material contained in this book.

The Publisher

Printed in Great Britain

Contents

Preface

This book addresses the need for nurses and midwives, both students and registered practitioners, to acquire the numerical skills and confidence necessary for safe practice. It is hoped that other health professionals will also derive benefit from this book. In addition to numerical skills, nurses will often be required to interpret clinical data from test results.

A number of publications have shown that the numerical skills of health professionals are often inadequate. Studies from the UK and beyond present a picture of lack of proficiency in mathematical calculation skills among both the student population and registered practitioners (Sabin 2002). It is not proposed to discuss in detail the reasons for this unfortunate situation, but a number of factors can be identified. Within both primary and secondary schools, pupils (especially girls) are often anxious about mathematics and in some schools there may be insufficient emphasis on basic mathematics. Teachers with the ability to present mathematics as a stimulating subject with a practical focus are difficult to recruit. The unpopularity of the subject, lack of confidence and pressures on time may also contribute to the difficulties experienced by students when they reach further or higher education.

A lack of proficiency in numerical skills may be compounded by pressures in the clinical environment, with an increased possibility of drug errors from miscalculation of dosages. Factors contributing to these pressures include the demands of a heavy workload, rapid development of medical technologies, expanding clinical roles and the use of information technology (IT).

Mistakes made in calculations are a significant cause of drug errors, especially in parenteral therapy (Taxis & Barber 2003), but it is important to set these errors in a wider context. Possible causes of drug errors, including calculation errors, and prevention strategies are well documented and are of increasing importance (Downie, Mackenzie & Williams 2003).

Overall, the impact of IT in both practice and teaching is essentially very positive and will become even more important in the years ahead. However, although computer technology is increasingly benefiting medicines management, the need for traditional numerical skills will remain. The safety of patients may be compromised if nurses rely solely on IT rather than on a sound understanding of basic arithmetic. The use of calculators to determine the volume or quantity of medication 'should not act as a substitute for arithmetical knowledge and skill' (NMC 2002 p. 7).

George Downie, Jean Mackenzie, Arthur Williams
Aberdeen, 2005

References

Downie G, Mackenzie J, Williams A 2003 Pharmacology and medicines management for nurses. 3rd edn. Churchill Livingstone, Edinburgh, pp 95–96.

NMC 2002 Guidelines for the administration of medicines. Nursing and Midwifery Council, London, p 7.

Sabin M 2002 Competence in practice-based calculation: issues for nursing education. Occasional Paper No. 3. LTSN-Centre for Health Sciences and Practice, London, p 17.

Taxis K, Barber N 2003 Ethnographic study of incidence and severity of intravenous errors. British Medical Journal 326: 684–686.

Acknowledgements

We are grateful for helpful advice from clinical colleagues Dorothy Dawson, Carol Doolan, Linda Park and Karen Watson, and able secretarial assistance from Lesley Anderson.

We are grateful to the following companies for permission to reproduce label artwork:

Abbott Laboratories for labels in Exercises 4.21, 4.44
Alpharma for Fig. 1.1, Labels 1.4, 3.1, 3.3, labels in Exercises 4.3, 4.4, 5.8
APS/Berk Pharmaceuticals for label in Exercise 4.13
AstraZeneca for label in Example 4.1
Bayer Healthcare for label in Exercise 4.37
Boehringer Ingelheim for labels in Exercises 4.33, 4.36, 4.56
Celltech Pharmaceuticals for labels in Exercises 5.1, 5.19
CP Pharmaceuticals for label in Exercise 4.28
Ferring Pharmaceuticals for label in Example 5.7
Forest Laboratories UK for label in Exercise 4.48
Generics (UK) for labels in Examples 4.4, 4.11, 4.13, Exercises 4.11, 4.12, 4.14, 4.16, 4.22, 4.27, 4.42
GlaxoSmithKline for labels in Examples 4.14, 5.1, Exercises 4.10, 4.39
Goldshield Pharmaceuticals for labels in Exercises 4.6, 5.3, 5.4, 5.5
Hameln Pharmaceuticals for labels in Exercises 5.6, 5.9, 5.18
Ivax Pharmaceuticals UK for Fig. 4.1, labels in Exercises 4.23, 4.25, 4.31
Janssen-Cilag for labels in Exercises 4.20, 4.26, 4.55
Leo Laboratories for labels in Example 4.12, Exercise 5.14
Lilly for label in Exercise 4.53
Link Pharmaceuticals for label in Exercise 4.30
Lundbeck for label in Exercise 4.38
Medeus Pharma for label in Example 4.7
Merck for label in Exercise 4.8
Organon Laboratories for labels in Exercises 4.5, 4.52
Pfizer for Labels 1.1, 1.3, labels in Exercises 4.2, 4.7, 4.9, 4.17, 4.29
Roche Products for labels in Examples 4.16, 5.2, 5.4, Exercises 4.47, 4.54, 5.17
Rosemont Pharmaceuticals for labels in Examples 4.2, 4.5, 4.15, Exercises 4.32, 4.34
Schering-Plough for label in Exercise 5.7
Sterwin Medicines for labels in Example 4.10, Exercise 4.41
The Wellcome Foundation for labels in Exercises 4.43, 4.51
Yamanouchi Pharma for label in Example 4.6

Introduction:
Why this book is needed

The administration of the right drug, in the right dose, to the right patient, at the right time is a cornerstone of nursing practice. To achieve the right dose, a drug calculation may be required.

When the subject of calculations is introduced for the first time into undergraduate courses, student nurses (and other health care professionals) often react in one of the following ways.

● 'I can't do them! I hated maths at school and I've never been good with figures.'
● 'I don't remember what I learned at school. I need help.'
● 'I can handle the theory, but how do I apply it?'

These reactions are frequently accompanied by expressions of understandable anxiety. To acquire the numeracy skills necessary for safe practice, it is important to acknowledge the level of assistance and practice you need.

On registration, nurses are deemed to be competent to practise in their chosen field and are accountable for their actions (and inactions). The role of mentor carries with it the added responsibilities of teaching and supervising students in administering medicines safely, including calculating what dose the patient is to be given. In specialist areas such as intensive care, oncology, etc., more advanced skills in calculations are likely to be required. At any level, registered nurses not only must be able to undertake calculations accurately but also require to know the normal dose range for the medicines they administer.

This publication is designed to enable nurses to achieve and maintain competence in calculating drug doses using different forms of medicines, and has been constructed in order to be:

Comprehensive   Achievable
Accessible   Teachable
Logical   Informative
Clinical   Original
Understandable   Non-threatening
Learnable   Systematic

It is emphasised that it is not a mathematical text. Rather, the approach throughout is one of promoting safe practice and reducing levels of anxiety.

CHAPTER **1**

Methods of expressing strengths of medicines

Learning outcomes

- Acquire a working knowledge of the metric system and the units derived from it
- Acquire a working knowledge of percentages
- Understand the basic structure and contents of the labels of medicines
- Appreciate what is considered 'good practice' in the expression of strengths of medicines

---

Metric system

The metric system is the standard system of weights (mass) and measures (volume) used today to express the strength of a medicine. The international system of units known as the SI system (Système International (d'Unités)) is the basis for the physical units used in practice. Other units derived from the basic metric units, for example, the millimole (mmol), are also widely used. The metric units shown below should always be used. Only standard abbreviations should be used; they are always singular, for example mg and not mgs.

Weight (mass)
1 kilogram (kg) = 1000 grams (g)
1 gram (g)   = 1000 milligrams (mg)
1 milligram (mg) = 1000 micrograms (do not abbreviate)
1 microgram   = 1000 nanograms (do not abbreviate)
1 nanogram   = 1000 picograms (do not abbreviate)

The units nanogram and picogram are seldom used in clinical practice.

Volume
1 litre   = 1000 millilitres (mL)
1 millilitre = 1000 microlitres (do not abbreviate)

The abbreviation 'mL' for millilitre is the printing convention used in the British National Formulary (BNF) (BMA and RPSGB latest issue) and is an acceptable abbreviation in clinical practice. The term litre is generally not abbreviated since it is safer to express volumes in millilitres.

Length

1 metre (m)   = 1000 millimetres (mm)
1 centimetre (cm) = 10 millimetres (mm)

The above units of mass and volume are used in expressing the strengths of medicines. Units of length are used in calculating doses of certain drugs (pp. 37–38).

The metric system is in daily use in the UK in all aspects of life. Its use in clinical work should not present any problems provided the guidance outlined below is followed:

● Learn and memorise the basic units and the relationship between them
● Take particular care with the placing of decimal points when writing decimal fractions
● Do not use such units as:
  • decilitre or centilitre
  • decigram or centigram
  as these may cause confusion

Other methods of expressing strengths of medicines

The need for a standard system of weight and volume is fundamental to the practice of medicine. There are occasions, however, when the strength of a medicine cannot be expressed directly in units of weight and volume.

For some products, the strength may be expressed as the number of parts (by weight) of the active ingredient (drug) contained in a given volume (mL). For example, the strength of epinephrine (adrenaline) injection is generally expressed as 1 in 1000 (1 g in 1000 mL) or 1 in 10000 (1 g in 10000 mL). The reasons for the use of this method of expressing strength are traditional. In practice, this method is more convenient, and probably safer, than the more usual system where the weight in a given volume is expressed as milligrams or micrograms per 1 mL. This is because a very wide range of dosage regimens of this potent drug is used in both paediatrics and adult medicine.

It is, however, important to understand how such an expression as 1 in 1000 can be converted to mg per mL or micrograms per mL. '1 in 1000' means that 1 g of the active drug is contained in 1000 mL of the injection solution, and

1 g in 1000 mL = 1000 mg in 1000 mL

Dividing by 1000, we get

1 mg in 1 mL

Converting mg to micrograms, we find that

1000 micrograms is contained in 1 mL

A similar approach can be followed to show that 1 mL of a 1 in 10000 solution contains 100 micrograms.

UNITS OF ACTIVITY

The strengths of some medicines obtained from natural biological (or semi-synthetic) sources are sometimes expressed in units of activity. Biological assays are used to standardise these products, since chemical methods cannot be applied. Examples of medicines where the strength is expressed in units are given in Table 1.1.

Since the drugs in Table 1.1 marked with an asterisk may be prescribed in units or micrograms, care is needed in interpreting prescriptions for these products (see BNF for strengths of available products).

Nurses will rarely be required to know the quantitative relationship between the units of activity and units of the metric system. The metric system equivalents for some units are given in the BNF, e.g. 1000 units is equivalent to 1 mg of dornase alfa. Local prescribing policies will normally determine how prescriptions should be written, i.e. in units of activity or units of mass. When prescribing drugs in units of activity, the word 'unit(s)' should not be abbreviated to 'u' since, if badly written, it may be mistaken for a zero, which could introduce a tenfold error.

Table 1.1 Examples of drugs expressed in units of activity

Drug group	Examples
Antibiotics	Bleomycin (cytotoxic antibiotic) Colistin Nystatin
Hormones	Calcitonin Gonadotrophins* Insulin Oxytocin Vasopressin
Immunological products	Immunoglobulins and interferons Immunological agents such as antisera
Vitamins	Vitamin A Vitamin D*
Other drugs	Dornase alfa* Epoetin alfa* Heparin

*May be expressed in units or micrograms

PERCENTAGES

The strength of most medicines is expressed as grams, milligrams, micrograms, etc. together with the volume in millilitres (mL) if it is a liquid medicine. For topical medicines and certain large volume injections, the strength of the ingredients is expressed as a percentage:

The term 'percentage' means 'parts per 100'
So, e.g., 10% means 10 parts per 100

For a mixture of two solids, the percentage is expressed as weight in weight (w/w), e.g.:

5% w/w means 5 g of an ingredient is present in 100 g of product

If, however, the preparation is a solid dissolved or suspended in a liquid, the percentage is expressed as weight in volume (w/v), e.g.:

5% w/v means 5 g of an ingredient is present in 100 mL of product

Where the product is a liquid diluted in another liquid, the percentage is expressed as volume in volume (v/v), e.g.:

5% v/v means 5 mL of an ingredient is present in 100 mL of product

In a few situations, a liquid is dispersed in a solid, in which case the percentage is expressed as volume in weight (v/w), e.g.:

5% v/w means 5 mL of an ingredient is present in 100 g of product

When considering a medicine, it is important to recognise that the active ingredient is evenly distributed throughout the product.

MOLARITY

The strength of the active (and other) ingredients of a medicine is expressed mainly by the use of the common metric units of weight and volume. Percentages are also widely used. Another important way of expressing the strength (concentration) of a medicine is the use of molarity. This can be a difficult concept for those who have not had a grounding in chemistry. In order to explain the concept of molarity, it is essential to refer to some basic chemistry:

● Each atom has an atomic weight, e.g. sodium 23, potassium 39, calcium 40 and chlorine 35.4
● Atoms combine to form a molecule, e.g. sodium (Na) combines with chlorine (Cl) to form sodium chloride. Sodium chloride has a molecular weight of 58.4 (the sum of the atomic weights)

Mole

The term 'mole' is defined as:

One mole of a drug weighs (in grams) the same as the relative molecular weight of that drug.

For sodium chloride, 1 mole weighs 58.4 g. A molar solution contains 1 mole in 1 litre of solvent, i.e.

58.4g sodium chloride in 1 litre

or in percentage terms

$$\frac{58.4}{1000} \times 100 = 5.84\% \text{ w/v}$$

Given that 1 mole of sodium chloride weighs 58.4g,

1 mole = 58.4 × 1000 mg

For practical purposes, millimoles (mmol), i.e. $\frac{1}{1000}$ mole, are used since this gives a more manageable unit.

$$1 \text{ mmol weighs } \frac{58.4 \times 1000 \text{mg}}{1000} = 58.4 \text{mg}$$

1 mmol of sodium chloride (58.4 mg) (chemical formula NaCl) contains 1 mmol Na^+ and 1 mmol Cl^-. The weight is the same for both ions.

A second example is magnesium chloride. The relative molecular mass (molecular weight) of magnesium chloride ($MgCl_2$ $6H_2O$) is 203.3 g, so

1 mole of the drug weighs 203.3 g, or 203.3 × 1000 mg

1 mmol of the drug weighs

$$\frac{203.3 \times 1000 \text{mg}}{1000} = 203.3 \text{mg}$$

From the chemical formula $MgCl_2$ $6H_2O$, it will be seen that, unlike sodium chloride, the weights containing 1 mmol of Mg^{2+} and Cl^- will not be the same, since the molecule contains two chlorine atoms:

1 mmol Mg^{2+} is contained in 203.3 mg

1 mmol Cl^- is contained in

$$\frac{203.3 \text{mg}}{2} = 101.7 \text{mg}$$

Micromole

This unit has the same relationship to the millimole as the microgram has to the milligram, i.e.

1 millimole = 1000 micromoles

Milliequivalents

The method of expressing the concentration of drugs and biochemical values in milliequivalents is not part of the SI system. Molarity is now the accepted system using units based on the mole, millimole and micromole.

Use of millimole in the labelling and prescribing of medicines

Nurses will generally not be required to calculate millimoles from first principles but will be required to administer drugs whose strength is expressed in mmol/litre, or mmol or micromol/mL. This applies especially to providing fluid replacement and correcting electrolyte imbalances. The strength of some oral preparations of, for example, calcium, potassium and sodium is often expressed in milligrams and millimoles per tablet.

Millimoles in clinical practice

Although drugs are not generally prescribed in molar doses, some drugs, such as lithium and potassium, may be prescribed in millimoles. Biochemical reports on drug concentrations will normally be given in millimoles per litre. Insulin is given according to blood glucose levels expressed in mmol litre to patients undergoing surgery (see BNF).

METRIC/IMPERIAL SYSTEM EQUIVALENTS

Although all medicine strengths are expressed using the metric system, there may be occasions where there is a need to make conversions, for example, of body weight, between the imperial (non-metric) system and the metric system. These conversions are included in the BNF.

Guidelines to good practice in the writing and use of metric weights and measures

- Take great care in the placing of decimal points
- *Always* write a zero before a decimal point for numbers less than 1, i.e. 0.1 (*never* .1)
- *Always* use approved abbreviations
- Take great care with fractions of a milligram. *Always* use micrograms, e.g. 250 micrograms (*never* 0.25 mg)
- *Always* use the exact weight or volume of the drug involved. The terms 'half a tablet' or 'half an ampoule' are open to misinterpretation and should not be used without further qualification
- Avoid, wherever possible, verbal communications regarding dosages. If these have to be used, speak slowly and clearly, repeating the message and documenting the information right away

Labels on medicine containers

Labels on medicine containers fulfil a number of functions that reflect the needs of all the professions involved in the manufacture, distribution and administration of medicines. The needs of patients in the community are being increasingly catered for as patient packs become the norm. For example, labels may show details of ingredients other than only the active drug.

The content of the label on a medicine container is controlled by various legal requirements defined in the EU directives. Requirements are specified for both the outer packaging and the inner foil or blister pack. Labelling on the outer package or on other packaging (e.g. bottle containing tablets) is more comprehensive than that on the inner (blister) pack.

The content of a typical label on an outer package is illustrated in Fig. 1.1. The focus for the nurse will be the name and strength of the product together with the expiry date. Batch numbers are used to identify the product in case of any faults which may require a product recall.

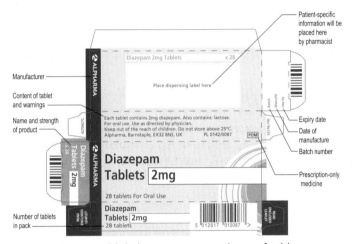

Figure 1.1 Typical label on an outer package of tablets.

The basic requirements for the main package are:

- Name of the medicinal product (proprietary name) followed by its common name (approved name)
- Statement of the active ingredients
- Formulation
- Any excipients
- Method of administration
- Warning to keep the product out of the reach of children
- Any special warning about the product itself
- Expiry date
- Special storage precautions
- Special precautions for disposal of unused product
- Name and address of holder of the product licence
- Product licence number
- Batch number
- In the case of self-medication, instructions for use

The following particulars must appear on blister or foil packs (The European Communities 1992):

● Name of the medicinal product followed by its common name
● Name of the holder of the product licence
● Expiry date
● Batch number

Not all the information provided by the label is of importance to the nurse administering the medicine. Interpretation of the label in relation to the prescription is dealt with on p. 27.

DRUG NAMES

Each label on a medicine container will generally show two names. For commercial reasons, the manufacturer often gives prominence to the proprietary name. Most prescribing policies require the use of the British Approved Name (BAN) or the Recommended International Non-proprietary Name (rINN).

Drug compounds used in the preparation of medicines

In order for a drug to be formulated into a medicine, it is often essential to use a compound of the drug that is soluble (and stable) in the preferred solvent, usually water. Many drugs are insoluble in water and must be chemically converted into a soluble form, such as a salt (morphine hydrochloride) or an ester (glyceryl trinitrate). Where it is not possible or desirable to prepare a soluble form of the drug, it will be formulated into a suspension.

Labels on pharmaceutical products will indicate the form in which the active drug is present. As an example, gentamicin injection contains 40 mg gentamicin as the sulphate.

Generally the compound used in the formulation will not be of major concern to the nurse, but in order to understand labels of medicines an appreciation of the principles involved is required.

There are special situations where the form of the drug is significant. Dexamethasone injection is available as 4 mg/mL, i.e. each mL contains 4 mg of dexamethasone as dexamethasone sodium phosphate. This should be taken into account when interpreting labels and prescriptions involving dexamethasone.

Questions about labels

The following exercises are designed to help in the reading and interpretation of labels. You may need to refer to the BNF in some instances.

Answers are on p. 145.

LABEL 1.1

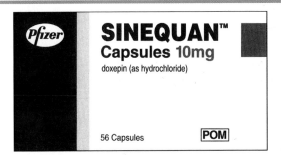

1. What is the approved name?
2. Could this medicine be bought from a pharmacy?
3. Is it acceptable to use a product labelled doxepin hydrochloride when doxepin has been prescribed?
4. The patient requires to take 40 mg daily. For how many weeks would a full pack last?

LABEL 1.2

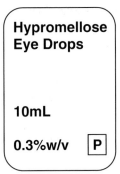

1. What does 0.3% w/v refer to?
2. What is the total volume of eye drops in an unopened bottle?
3. Apart from the standard advice given on all medicine labels, what special advice is given for eye drops?
4. What does P signify?

LABEL 1.3

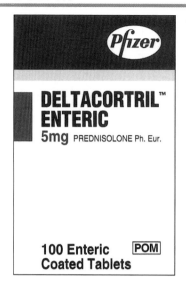

1. What does ™ stand for?
2. What is meant by 'enteric coated'?
3. What is meant by the 'proprietary' name?
4. What does Ph. Eur. mean?
5. What additional information should you make the patient aware of relating to this product?

LABEL 1.4

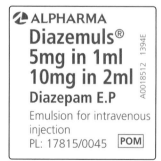

1. What does ® signify?
2. Would you administer this product to a patient with a known allergy to eggs?
3. What does PL stand for?
4. By what route would this product be administered?

REFERENCES

BMA and RPSGB (latest issue) British National Formulary. British Medical Association and Royal Pharmaceutical Society of Great Britain, London.

The European Communities (Designation) (No. 2) Order 1992. Statutory Instrument 1992 No. 1711.

CHAPTER 2

Essential arithmetic

Learning outcomes

- Understand the broad principles of arithmetic
- Understand what is meant by fractions and decimals
- Be able to simplify fractions; change decimals to fractions; change fractions to decimals
- Understand and be able to use proportion
- Understand the concept of percentages

Numerical skills required by nurses

In order to accurately calculate drug doses and interpret data in other health care situations, it is essential to have certain arithmetical skills. On most occasions, the skills required are not complex; in fact, they are relatively straightforward. The skills routinely needed, either singly or in combination, are as follows (Sabin 2002, adapted from Hilton 1999):

- Adding*
- Subtracting*
- Multiplying*
- Dividing*
- Simplifying fractions
- Changing decimals to fractions
- Changing fractions to decimals
- Using proportion
- Using percentages

(*The assumption is made that the reader is competent in these skills.)

Fundamental arithmetical principles

NUMBERS

- All numbers are either even numbers or odd numbers
- Even numbers (2, 4, 6, 8, etc.) can all be divided by 2 to leave a whole number

- Odd numbers (1, 3, 5, 7, etc.) cannot be divided by 2 to leave a whole number
- Any number ending in either a 5 or a zero can be divided by 5

EXPRESSING FIGURES

When making any type of calculation, there may be times when you need to express a number in a way that will assist you. Take any number, let's say 6.

- The figure 6 can be expressed as $^6/_1$ without altering the fact that it is 6
- The figure 6 can also be expressed as 6.0000 without altering the fact that it is 6
- Any number of zeros can be placed after the decimal point; the number will still be valued as 6

Great care is needed when working with very large numbers (e.g. 100000; 250000). It is no longer common to see in print the use of commas to signify thousands (e.g. 100,000; 250,000). It *is* advisable, however, to use commas when working on paper to ensure you have the right number of zeros.

Explaining fractions and decimals

The word fraction means a 'fragment of something'.

The word decimal means 'based on the number ten'.

Fractions may be expressed in two ways:

- as a vulgar fraction (e.g. $^3/_5$, often simply referred to as a 'fraction')
- as a decimal fraction (e.g. 0.6, often simply referred to as a 'decimal')

'Fractions' and 'decimals' are two ways of expressing a part of something. There will of course be times when the fraction or the decimal will be added to a whole number, e.g. $1\frac{1}{4}$, 1.25.

FRACTIONS

'Fractions' are commonly used in everyday life, e.g.,

- $\frac{1}{2}$ the class
- $\frac{1}{4}$ of an apple
- $4\frac{1}{2}$ working days (whole number plus a fraction)

but are less often used for precise measurement.

A fraction for our purposes is formed when a number is placed above another number and the two numbers are separated by a dividing line, e.g.,

$^3/_5$, $^5/_5$, $^8/_5$ are all fractions

The number above the line is known as the numerator; the number below the line is the denominator. If the two numbers are the same, they will cancel each other out to become one. So,

$^5/_5 = 1$ (five fifths is the whole)

If the number above the line is less than the number below the line, the fraction is always less than one. So,

$^3/_5 < 1$ (three fifths is less than the whole)

If the number above the line is more than the number below the line, the fraction must be *more* than one. So,

$^8/_5 > 1$ (eight fifths, or $1^3/_5$, is more than the whole)

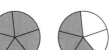

DECIMALS

'Decimals' are used in the metric system and are measured in tenths, e.g.,

● 28.3 g jar of marmalade $(28 + ^3/_{10}$ g)
● 304.8 mm length of wood $(304 + ^8/_{10}$ mm)
● 3.6 kg baby $(3 + ^6/_{10}$ kg)

The decimal point is placed before the decimal fraction.

Quantities that are less than one should normally be written as a whole number of the next unit down, e.g.,

● 750 mg rather than 0.75 g
● 125 micrograms and not 0.125 mg

Never start a figure with a decimal point. For example, always write 0.6 and *not* .6. In this case, no doubt you can detect the decimal point but there may be times when the 'decimal point' is a blob of ink on the page!

When a fraction is expressed in decimal form:

● Any number starting with '0.' must be less than one (e.g. 0.6)
● The quantity one is expressed as 1
● Any number more than one is either a whole number or a whole number plus a decimal fraction (e.g. 1.6)

These figures can be illustrated on a scale, as in Fig. 2.1.

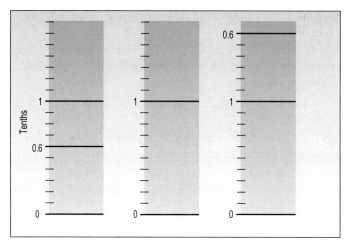

Figure 2.1 Decimal scale.

Simplifying fractions (cancelling down)

When using fractions, it is always best to simplify them as far as possible, since it is easier (and safer) to work with smaller figures than with bigger ones. For example, $^{750}/_{250}$ could be immediately simplified by removing the zeros to give $^{75}/_{25}$, making sure of course to delete the same number of zeros above and below the line. The fraction could then be simplified by dividing the numbers above and below the line by 25 to give

$$^3/_1 = 3$$

Taking another example of a calculation which involves a fraction,

$$^{15}/_{20} \times 2$$

The 15 is to be *divided* by the 20. Another way of putting this is to say '20 into 15'. The result is then to be multiplied by 2.

However, it could be made easier if we were to simplify this fraction first by saying

$$^{15}/_{20} \times 2 \text{ is the same as } ^{15}/_{20} \times ^2/_1$$

You now have the choice of :

● either simplifying the 15 and the 20 (directly)
● or simplifying the 2 and the 20 (diagonally)

It does not matter which of these options you use or in what order. The 15 and the 1 cannot be further simplified.

Let's start by cancelling above and directly below the line. Both the 15 and the 20 can be divided by 5, so

$$\frac{^{3}\cancel{15}}{\cancel{20}_{4}} \times \frac{2}{\cancel{1}} = \frac{3}{4} \times \frac{2}{\cancel{1}}$$

Then we can simplify again by cancelling above and diagonally below the line. Both the 2 and the 4 can be divided by 2, so

$$\frac{3}{\cancel{4}_{2}} \times \frac{\cancel{2}^{1}}{\cancel{1}} = \frac{3}{2} \times \frac{\cancel{1}}{1}$$
$$= \frac{3}{2}$$

Changing fractions to decimals

At times, it may be necessary to change your answer from a fraction to a decimal, e.g. prior to drawing up a volume of drug into a syringe.

EXAMPLE

$\frac{3}{5}$ is the same as saying 3 is to be divided by 5. This may be represented as

either $5\overline{)3}$ *or* $5\overline{)3}$

which is the same as $5\overline{)3.0}$ *or* $5\overline{)3.0}$

which works out as $5\overline{)3.^{3}0}$ *or* $\dfrac{0.6}{5\overline{)3.^{3}0}}$
0.6

The answer, either way, is 0.6.

Here are some examples of fractions. See if you can change them into decimals.

(a) $\frac{3}{4}$
(b) $\frac{3}{2}$
(c) $\frac{1}{4}$
(d) $\frac{1}{10}$
(e) $\frac{2}{5}$

Answers to these are on p. 146.

Changing decimals to fractions

As part of the process of working out a drug calculation, you will at times want to change a decimal into a fraction.

EXAMPLE

0.6 is to be converted to a fraction.

0.6 is the same as $\frac{0.6}{1}$

which is the same as $\frac{0.6}{1.0}$

which is the some as $\frac{0.\overset{\frown}{6}}{1.\overset{\frown}{0}}$

which becomes $\frac{6}{10}$

which cancels down to $\frac{3}{5}$

Here are some more decimals for you to change into fractions.

(a) 0.1
(b) 0.5
(c) 0.25
(d) 0.75
(e) 0.2

Answers to these are on p. 146.

Acceptable manipulation of figures

When you have a fraction, for example $\frac{6}{10}$, you can divide the figure above the line and the figure below the line by the same number without fundamentally altering the fraction. Since both 6 and 10 are divisible by 2,

$$\frac{6}{10} = \frac{3}{5}$$

The fraction $\frac{6}{10}$ has been simplified, but the relationship between the two figures has not changed.

If the fraction is made up of numbers that contain a decimal point, such as $\frac{2.5}{7.5}$, it is acceptable to move the decimal points, provided you move them *the same number of places in the same direction, above the line and below the line*. It is always better to create a whole number wherever possible anyway. This can only ever be done by moving the decimal point to the *right*. So, to take the example of $\frac{2.5}{7.5}$, if we move both points one place to the right, we get

$25/_{75}$ (which can be simplified)

$$= \frac{1 \text{ (i.e. 25 divided by 25)}}{3 \text{ (i.e. 75 divided by 25)}}$$

If you want to change one side of an equation you must do *exactly the same* to the other side, e.g.:

$1\,g = 1000\,mg$

So

$0.5\,g = 500\,mg$ (both sides divided by 2)

and

$0.1\,g = 100\,mg$ (both sides divided by 5)

Sometimes you arrive at an answer that you cannot finish because the last digit repeats itself, e.g.:

6.3333 (rep.)
6.6666 (rep.)

In medicines for *adults:*

Any number beyond the decimal point that is *less* than in this case 6.5 would be rounded *down* to the nearest whole number, 6

Any number beyond the decimal point that is *greater* than 6.5 would be rounded *up* to the nearest whole number, 7

In medicines for *neonates and children:*

It is advisable to seek advice on each occasion that this situation arises.

Simple proportion

'Proportion' means the relation of one thing to another in magnitude. In arithmetic, it is referred to as simple proportion.

For example, you need 2500 sheets of photocopying paper, which is supplied in packets of 500 sheets.

From the above information, it is clear that *more* than one packet is required.

There is a direct numerical (proportional) relationship between the *number of sheets* required and the *number of packets* required. This can be expressed as a simple equation. If x is the number of packets required:

$$x = \frac{\text{Total number of sheets required}}{\text{Number of sheets per packet}}$$

$$x = \frac{2500}{500}$$

$$x = 5$$

You will need 5 packets.

Or you can say:

500 sheets = 1 packet
2500 sheets = x packets

The proportions of sheets and packets will be equal:

$$\frac{500}{2500} = \frac{1}{x}$$

Cross multiply:

$$500x = 1 \times 2500$$
$$x = \frac{1 \times 2500}{500}$$
$$x = 5$$

You will need 5 packets.

A more complex example: you are organising a fundraising party. 250 people wish to attend. Your budget indicates that 200 guests would cost £2000. You need to know what it would cost to cater for 250 people.

From the above information, it is clear that the cost will be *more* than £2000.

There is a direct numerical (proportional) relationship between the *cost of 200 guests* and the *cost of 250 guests*. This can be expressed as a simple equation. If x is the cost (£) of 250 guests:

$$x = \text{Cost of 200 guests} \times \frac{250}{200}$$
$$= 2000 \times \frac{250}{200}$$
$$= 10 \times 250$$
$$= £2500$$

Or, because the proportions of guests and costs will be equal:

$$\frac{200}{250} = \frac{2000}{x}$$

Cross multiply:

$$200x = 250 \times 2000$$
$$x = \frac{250 \times 2000}{200}$$
$$x = 10 \times 250$$
$$x = £2500$$

In the previous examples, we wanted to find quantities greater than the basic number given (one packet of paper in the first example and £2000 in the second). Now we will apply the same approach to find a quantity that is *less* than the basic number given.

The cost of renting an audio/visual system is £250 a year. You want to work out the cost for a 10-week period.

It is clear that the cost for a 10-week period will be less than £250. One year = 52 weeks, so, if x is the cost of renting for a 10-week period:

$x = $ Cost (£) of 1 year's rental $\times {}^{10}\!/_{52}$

$x = 250 \times \dfrac{10}{52}$

$x = $ approx. £48

Or, because the proportions of weeks and costs will be equal:

$$\frac{10}{52} = \frac{x}{250}$$

Cross multiply:

$10 \times 250 = 52x$

$$x = \frac{10 \times 250}{52}$$

$$= \text{approx. } £48$$

Simple proportion is the basis from which the formula used to calculate a drug dose is derived (see p. 33).

Percentages

A percentage is written as 50%, 29%, 94%, etc. The term percentage means 'parts per 100' and for the purpose of a calculation can be expressed as the number preceding the % sign divided by 100, i.e. its value expressed in hundredths. So,

50% is the same as ${}^{50}\!/_{100}$
29% is the same as ${}^{29}\!/_{100}$
94% is the same as ${}^{94}\!/_{100}$

If 50% of a group of workers carry a packed lunch, that means ${}^{50}\!/_{100}$ do so, which is half the group. We do not know the size of the group but we know that half of them carry a packed lunch.

To take another example, if 39% out of a group of 700 patients were said to be in favour of open visiting, the actual number of patients in favour could be calculated as follows:

$$\frac{39}{100} \times 700 = 273$$

That means that 273 patients are said to be in favour of open visiting.

As a final example, you know that out of a class of 168 students, 126 carry a mobile phone. That may be expressed as $^{126}/_{168}$. To obtain the percentage who carry a mobile phone, $^{126}/_{168}$ must be multiplied by 100:

$$\frac{126}{168} \times 100 = \frac{3}{4} \times 100$$
$$= \frac{300}{4}$$
$$= 75$$

75% of the class carry a mobile phone.

Summary

There are a number of ways of working out arithmetical problems. It does not matter a bit which method you use; use the one you are most comfortable with. What *does* matter is that your method helps you reach the right answer every time.

Arithmetic is an exact science. A careless arithmetical slip could have disastrous consequences. The secret is to take your time and stick to the rules. Because of their critical importance, the key points highlighted in this chapter are listed below.

● Any number can be placed above a one without changing its value, e.g.

125 is the same as $^{125}/_1$

● Any number can have a decimal point and any number of zeros added to it without changing its value, e.g.

125 is the same as 125.000000

● It is always safer to work in whole numbers whenever possible
● When simplifying a vulgar fraction, you can cancel directly 'up and down' or 'diagonally'
● When moving decimal points in a fraction, the points must be moved the same number of places in the same direction both above and below the line
● In a vulgar fraction, the value of the number above the line tells you whether you are dealing with more than one or less than one, e.g. $\frac{3}{4}$ is less than $\frac{4}{3}$

If you have forgotten your multiplication tables, now is the time to brush them up. Leave your calculator aside and pull out a piece of paper and a pencil. With guidance, many students succeed in carrying out quite intricate manoeuvres when calculating drug dosages. What often lets them down is whether or not they know '2 twos are 4; 2 threes are 6; 2 fours are 8', etc. No amount of training in drug calculations will suffice unless these basic skills are learned and practised.

The next chapter describes how to do a drug calculation, where arithmetical skills will be brought to bear on this vitally important aspect of patient care.

REFERENCES

Sabin M 2002 Competence in practice-based calculation: issues for nursing education. Occasional Paper No. 3 LTSN-Centre for Health Sciences and Practice, London, p. 17.

CHAPTER **3**
How to do a drug calculation

Learning outcomes

- Recognise what constitutes a valid prescription
- Be able to interpret the information on a medicine label
- Understand the relationship between the quantitative details on the prescription and the quantitative details on the medicine label
- Recognise whether or not a calculation is required
- Understand the workings of calculations of varying levels of difficulty
- Select, understand and be able to use a method of calculating drug doses with which you are comfortable
- Be able to calculate drug doses based on body weight and body surface area (adults and children)
- Have an appreciation of the effects of a drug dose on different patients' weights
- Be aware that some solutions may require to be diluted before use

Relating prescription information to the label on the medicine container

THE PRESCRIPTION

A prescription may be defined as an authorised health professional's written or computer-generated instruction for the composition and use of a medicine. A valid prescription must meet current legal requirements.

The prescription is the first thing to look at. All prescriptions must clearly indicate the details required to identify the patient. In hospital practice, every prescription must include six key items. These are:

- date
- medicine
- dose
- route
- time(s) or frequency of administration
- prescriber's signature, in full, for each medicine prescribed

If any of the six key items is missing or unclear, *do not* proceed. The prescription must be referred back to the prescriber for amendment.

The patient's height and weight should also appear on the prescription sheet, where the dose is dependent on body weight or body surface area (see p. 36).

THE LABEL

The term 'label' is used in this text to mean the information relevant to the particular product, which with modern packaging is often integral to the package.

When reading the label on the medicine container, particular attention should be paid to the following points:

● Labels are prepared with various needs in mind; doctors, pharmacists, nurses and patients have their own information requirements. You must therefore get used to selecting the information you need from the label. Labels may vary in the way they are set out and so you may find that in practice you have to examine all sides of the container to get the information you require (see p. 7)
● Look at how the dose on the label is expressed. The quantity of drug in each 'item' in the pack or bottle must be identified. 'Item' is being used here to mean, for example, one tablet, one capsule, so many millilitres of liquid, one suppository, one inhalation

For example, the label may state:

```
Diazepam Tablets
2 mg
```

This means that each tablet contains 2 mg of active drug; or it may state:

```
Flucloxacillin Syrup
250 mg in 5 mL
```

This means that every 5 mL measured from the bottle (after it has been shaken) contains 250 mg of active drug.

The exception to this rule is a compound medicine (generally a solid form of a medicine). An example of a label of a compound might be:

```
Co-dydramol Tablets
Each containing:
dihydrocodeine tartrate 10 mg
and  paracetamol 500 mg
```

There is only one product known as co-dydramol and so it is acceptable for the prescription simply to state CO-DYDRAMOL 2 tablets (or 2 tab). That is precisely what the patient should get.

Note, however, that some compound preparations contain different strengths of active ingredients. For example, a label may state:

Co-amilofruse 2.5/20 Tablets
Each tablet contains:
amiloride hydrochloride 2.5 mg
and furosemide 20 mg

As the name suggests, co-amilofruse is a compound made up of amiloride and furosemide and in this example would appear on a prescription as co-amilofruse 2.5/20. Co-amilofruse tablets are also available in 5/40 and 10/80 strengths, and so it is essential to differentiate between the strengths before giving the dose.

RELATING DETAILS ON THE LABEL TO THE PRESCRIPTION

Every time (even in an emergency) a medicine is to be administered, no matter who is involved, there is a recognised procedure to be followed. The steps of this process are:

1. Read the details on the prescription
2. Read the details on the medicine label
3. Read the prescription again

In this way, the details on the one are being *compared* with the details on the other and thus it can be established whether the correct strength (or combination of strengths) of preparation has been selected and whether a calculation is required.

Particular points to note when examining the details on the label and starting to work out what the patient will be given are as follows:

● Medicines are often available in different strengths in order to meet most clinical needs without the necessity for complex calculations. For example,

Diazepam tablets	2 mg	5 mg	10 mg
Levothyroxine tablets	25 micrograms	50 micrograms	100 micrograms
Warfarin tablets	1 mg	3 mg	5 mg

Select the strength(s) which will result in the patient receiving the correct dose with the minimum number of tablets

● Particular care is needed when working with units that are less than a milligram, such as micrograms and nanograms. Dosages given in micrograms and nanograms indicate that very little of the drug is required to provide a therapeutic effect

● When dealing with liquid medicines, remember to look on the label for the strength of the drug (e.g. 500 mg) and the volume in which it is contained (e.g. 5 mL)

● Whenever possible, try to avoid having to divide a tablet to get the required dose. In some cases, however, this cannot be avoided. Only attempt to split a tablet if it is scored. *Never* try to split a coated tablet as this will defeat the purpose of the coating and would introduce an inaccuracy. Where a tablet splitter is available, use it. If there is difficulty, ask the pharmacist – he/she may be able to provide an alternative formulation. Similarly, capsules should not be opened unless prescribed in this way

● The utmost care is required when dealing with doses involving thousands of units of activity (e.g. nystatin 100,000 units/mL). As always, carefully read the prescription and the label, paying particular attention to the number of zeros

● If it appears that a dose has to be made up of several tablets or ampoules, check that all is in order. Your patient will not mind waiting a little longer if this means he/she gets the correct dose

IS A CALCULATION NECESSARY?

Prior to the administration of a medicine, it is always important to understand fully how the information on the label of the medicine container relates to the prescription. You may find that a calculation of the dose the patient is to receive is not required. If the strength of the available product exactly matches the prescribed dose, there is no need to make a calculation.

In the case of a compound preparation, i.e. a product containing more than one active ingredient, the exact amount to be given to the patient (e.g. 2 tablets in the case of a solid, 15 mL for a liquid) will be stated on the prescription and so again no calculation is needed. It is reassuring to know too that, wherever possible, the pharmacist will supply the medicine in the most appropriate form, thus reducing the need for a calculation.

In deciding whether or not there is a need to make a calculation, the following steps should be taken prior to administering the medicine:

● Ensure the prescription is clearly written
● Ensure the strength of the medicine, whether in solid or liquid form, is clearly shown. If there are any queries, they should be discussed with a senior colleague
● Check that the units of strength on the prescription match the units of strength on the label. For example, do not accept a prescription where the dose is given as a decimal fraction of a milligram when the strength on the label is expressed in micrograms. A quantity that is less than 1 mg should be written in micrograms, e.g. 250 micrograms and not 0.25 mg. Similarly, a quantity less than 1 microgram should be expressed in nanograms

WHERE A CALCULATION IS REQUIRED

Decide on a method for making the calculation with which you are comfortable (see pp. 30, 33).

- It is often very helpful at this stage to consider whether the total quantity required by the patient will be more than or less than what is contained in a single unit of the medicine. For example:

Dose prescribed   10 mg
Strength available   20 mg/2 mL

The answer *must* be less than 2 mL

- Make the calculation mentally or in the written form. Where a check to the answer is required or when making complex calculations, the assistance of a calculator may be appropriate (see p. 40)
- Where a calculation results in a quantity such as 1.78 mg or 2.333 mL, it will not be possible to administer these exact doses using normal clinical equipment. The decision to round up or down will be dependent on clinical factors such as the nature of the drug and the patient's weight, age and clinical condition
- Do not hesitate to ask a second nurse (or other competent colleague) to check your answer if you need reassurance
- Only proceed to give the medicine when you feel confident. Remember that, as with all your professional practice, you should be prepared to account for (i.e. explain, justify) your actions if required (NMC 2002)

With experience, you will find that it is unnecessary to go painstakingly through the steps outlined above prior to each medicine administration since, with practice, they will come naturally.

It is of the utmost importance that the principles involved are fully understood and upheld at all times. Discussion of these principles may be found as follows:

- Use of SI units (pp. 1–2)
- Basic arithmetic (p. 13)
- Interpretation of a prescription (p. 25)
- Interpretation of a label (p. 26)

LEVEL OF CALCULATION REQUIRED

Where a calculation is necessary, it can be considered to be at one of four levels. These levels are arbitrary and make no distinction between oral and parenteral therapy but are based on a risk assessment approach, i.e. the more complex the calculation, the greater the risk of error. It should be noted that all drug calculations are based on the same overall approach, i.e. a comparison between the dose to be given and the product available.

Level I. Straightforward calculations using elementary arithmetic
Level II. Based on the use of proportion but may involve different units such as milligrams and micrograms, and decimal fractions

Level III. Similar to Level II but may require the use of micrograms, nanograms, units of activity and millimoles. Non-standard products may be involved

Level IV. Involves a series of stages such as those where the dose is determined by body weight or body surface area. Of particular importance in parenteral therapy, especially where the dilution of a concentrated solution is involved

By far the majority of calculations are at Levels I and II. Whatever the level of the calculation, care is essential. It may be necessary to slow down, to check your answer and to ask a colleague to make an independent calculation, if possible by another method, so that you are quite certain before proceeding. Normally, such action is not needed but, when it is required, it should be considered as a safe and sensible precaution and in no sense a sign of inadequacy or cause for embarrassment.

Methods used to calculate drug doses

All drug calculations are based on a clear understanding of essential arithmetic and a sound working knowledge of the metric system. The ability to solve complex problems is not required but absolute accuracy is essential.

Two possible approaches may be used when making a calculation; the method used is often a matter of personal choice. It is important to use a method with which you are comfortable. Both methods described below can be used for all levels of calculations (see pp. 29–30) and one method can be used to check the other.

METHOD 1: USING THE GIVEN INFORMATION

This method does not require the use of a formula but is based on using the information regarding the dose of the drug on the prescription and the strength of the drug as given by the label on the medicine container. It does require a logical, stepwise approach. A number of examples of the use of this method are given below. Examples drawn from clinical practice are given in Chapters 4 and 5.

In most cases, drug calculations pose the same question for the nurse, i.e. how to obtain the dose prescribed from the particular dosage form (tablet, capsule, liquid) in the strength available.

Examples using solid dose medicines are generally very straightforward. In many cases, the required calculation can be carried out mentally, but it is important to understand the principles involved since these form the basis of more complex calculations.

Example 1

A patient is prescribed a dose of 20 mg of a drug orally	The tablets available each contain 10 mg of the drug

The number of tablets needed to make up the dose is calculated by comparing the strength of the available tablet with the dose prescribed. This can be expressed simply, as a fraction:

$$\frac{\text{Dose required}}{\text{Strength of available tablet}} = \frac{20\,mg}{10\,mg}$$

$$= 2$$

The prescribed dose is contained in 2 tablets.

Example 2

The patient is prescribed a 1 g dose of a drug orally

The tablets available contain 500 mg of the drug

Again a comparison is made between the dose prescribed and the strength of the available tablet. Each strength must be expressed in the same units, in this case milligrams, when making the calculation. So, as 1 g = 1000 mg,

$$\frac{\text{Dose required}}{\text{Strength of available tablet}} = \frac{1000\,mg}{500\,mg}$$

$$= 2$$

The prescribed dose is contained in 2 tablets.

Example 3

In this Example, and Examples 4, 5 and 6, the medicine available is in the form of a liquid and it is necessary to take this into account when making the calculation.

The sign ≡ is used to indicate that the dose (weight) and volume containing that dose are equivalent.

The patient is prescribed 400 mg of a drug orally

The drug is available as a syrup containing 500 mg of the drug in 5 mL

In order to make a comparison between the prescribed dose and the strength of the available product, it is useful to calculate the amount of drug contained in 1 mL of syrup. From the given information,

500 mg ≡ 5 mL

So dividing by 5,

100 mg ≡ 1 mL

Then

$$\frac{\text{Dose required (mg)}}{\text{Strength of available product (mg per mL)}} = \frac{\text{Number of mL of product}}{\text{to give required dose}}$$

$$\frac{400\,mg}{100\,mg} = 4\,mL$$

The prescribed dose is contained in 4 mL of syrup.

Example 4

This example involves the use of micrograms.

The patient is prescribed 20 micrograms of a drug orally

The drug is available as a liquid containing 35 micrograms in 5 mL

To make the comparison, first calculate the amount of drug contained in 1 mL of liquid. From the given information,

35 micrograms ≡ 5 mL

So dividing by 5,

7 micrograms ≡ 1 mL

Making the comparison,

$$\frac{\text{Dose required (micrograms)}}{\text{Strength of available product (micrograms/mL)}} = \frac{\text{Number of mL of product}}{\text{to give required dose}}$$

$$= {}^{20}\!/_7 \text{ mL}$$

This gives, after cancelling down, 2.857 mL. In practice, this would be rounded up to 2.86 mL.

The prescribed dose is contained in 2.86 mL.

Example 5

The patient is prescribed 500 micrograms by intramuscular injection

The drug is available as a 1 in 1000 solution (in 1 mL ampoules)

The drug is available as a 1 in 1000 solution. This is the same as saying that 1 gram of the drug is contained in 1000 mL of solution, i.e.

1 g ≡ 1000 mL

Converting 1 g to milligrams,

1000 mg ≡ 1000 mL

Dividing by 1000 to give mg/mL,

1 mg ≡ 1 mL

Converting 1 mg to micrograms,

1000 micrograms ≡ 1 mL

The volume required for the prescribed dose (in mL) is obtained by making the comparison

$$\frac{\text{Dose required (micrograms)}}{\text{Strength of available product (micrograms/mL)}} = \frac{500}{1000}$$

$$= 0.5 \text{ mL}$$

The prescribed dose is contained in 0.5 mL of the available solution.

METHOD 2: USING THE GIVEN INFORMATION IN A FORMULA

The second approach to drug calculations is based on the use of a formula which is based on proportion (see p. 19). Essentially, this method is similar to Method 1 but it may be preferred because of ease of use.

If the required dose is a simple multiple of the strength of the dosage form (as in Examples 1 and 2), there is no need to use a formula. The required calculation can be done mentally, although a formula may be used if preferred. Again the approach is essentially a comparison between the dose required and the strength of the available product.

$$\text{Number of tablets needed for use} = \frac{\text{Dose required in mg}}{\text{Dosage available per tablet in mg}} \times 1 \text{ tablet}$$

As an aide memoire, this can be expressed as

$$\frac{\text{Want (mg)}}{\text{Got (mg)}} \times 1 \text{ tablet} = \text{No. of tablets to make up the required dose}$$

Example 6

The patient is prescribed a dose of 20 mg orally

The tablets available each contain 10 mg of the drug

$$\text{No. of tablets to make up the dose} = \frac{\text{Want}}{\text{Got}} \times 1 \text{ tablet}$$
$$= \frac{20 \text{ mg}}{10 \text{ mg}} \times 1$$
$$= 2$$

The prescribed dose is contained in 2 tablets.

Example 7

The patient is prescribed a dose of 1 g (1000 mg) of a drug orally

The tablets available contain 500 mg of the drug

Applying the formula,

$$\text{No. of tablets to make up the dose} = \frac{\text{Want}}{\text{Got}} \times 1 \text{ tablet}$$
$$= \frac{1000 \text{ mg}}{500 \text{ mg}} \times 1$$
$$= 2$$

The prescribed dose is contained in 2 tablets.

Example 8

The patient is prescribed 400 mg of a drug orally	The drug is available as a syrup containing 500 mg of the drug in 5 mL

This example involves the use of a liquid medicine and therefore it is necessary to take this into account in the calculation. The formula now includes the volume of product containing the dosage available.

Applying the formula,

$$\frac{\text{Dose required (mg)}}{\text{Dosage available (mg)}} \times \text{Volume containing available dose (mL)}$$
$$= \text{Volume containing the required dose (mL)}$$

or

$$\frac{\text{Want (mg)}}{\text{Got (mg)}} \times \text{Volume containing got (mL)} = \text{Volume containing the required dose (mL)}$$

$$\frac{400\,\text{mg}}{500\,\text{mg}} \times 5\,\text{mL} = 4\,\text{mL}$$

The prescribed dose is contained in 4 mL of syrup.

Example 9

This example involves the use of micrograms.

The patient is prescribed 20 micrograms of a drug	The drug is available as a liquid containing 35 micrograms in 5 mL

Applying the formula, with micrograms replacing mg as the units to be used,

$$\frac{\text{Want (micrograms)}}{\text{Got (micrograms)}} \times \text{Volume containing got (mL)} = \text{Volume containing required dose (mL)}$$

$$\frac{20\,\text{micrograms}}{35\,\text{micrograms}} \times 5\,\text{mL} = \frac{20}{7}$$
$$= 2.857\,\text{mL}$$

The prescribed dose is contained in 2.857 mL. This dose would normally be rounded up to 2.86 mL (see p. 19).

Example 10

This example again involves the use of micrograms but the route of administration is by injection. The fact that this is a parenteral medicine does not affect the method used to calculate the dose.

The patient is prescribed 500 micrograms by intramuscular injection	The drug is available as a 1 in 1000 solution (in 1 mL ampoules)

Since the strength of the solution is expressed as '1 in 1000' it is necessary to convert this into micrograms per 1 mL in order that the formula can be applied.

1 in 1000 is the same as saying 1 g of drug is contained in 1000 mL of solution, i.e.

$$1 g \equiv 1000 \, mL$$

Converting to milligrams,

$$1000 \, mg \equiv 1000 \, mL$$

Dividing by 1000 to give mg/mL,

$$1 \, mg \equiv 1 \, mL$$

Converting to micrograms,

$$1000 \text{ micrograms} \equiv 1 \, mL$$

So, applying the formula,

$$\frac{\text{Want (micrograms)}}{\text{Got (micrograms)}} \times \text{Volume containing got (mL)} = \frac{\text{Volume containing}}{\text{required dose (mL)}}$$

$$\frac{500 \text{ micrograms}}{1000 \text{ micrograms}} \times 1 mL = 0.5 \, mL$$

The prescribed dose is contained in 0.5 mL solution.

The advantages and disadvantages of each calculation method are summarised in Table 3.1.

Each method requires the same basic competencies, namely, the ability to do essential arithmetic and a good working knowledge of the metric system.

In the worked examples in Chapters 4 and 5, 'using the given information' (Method 1) is used for oral solid dose forms (tablets and capsules) and the 'formula method' (Method 2) is used for liquid medicines (oral and injection).

Table 3.1 Advantages and disadvantages of two methods of calculating drug doses

Method 1: Using given information	Method 2: Using given information in a formula
Advantages	**Advantages**
Logical and stepwise	Easy to apply in busy working situation
Disadvantages	**Disadvantages**
More time-consuming than formula method A number of lines of working could introduce errors	Incorrect figures may be inserted into the formula, leading to errors May lead to complacency and lack of understanding of basic principles Nurses may be put off by the idea of a formula

Drug doses based on body weight and body surface area (BSA)

Calculation of doses based on body weight or BSA may be classed as Level IV, since there are at least two stages involved.

DRUG DOSES BASED ON BODY WEIGHT (ADULTS)

A number of drugs, notably cytotoxic drugs, are given in doses which are calculated according to body weight. This method of dosage determination is necessary in order to minimise adverse reactions, since the dose is 'tailored' to the needs of the individual patient. Examples of drugs given in doses related to body weight are busulfan and chlorambucil.

Example 1

The daily dose of busulfan (for the induction of remission in the treatment of chronic myeloid leukaemia) is 60 micrograms per kg up to a maximum of 4 mg daily. The patient's weight is 63.5 kg.

The calculation involves multiplying the patient's weight by the dose per kg:

63.5 kg × 60 micrograms per kg = 3810 micrograms

The patient would receive 3.81 mg daily.

Example 2

The dose of chlorambucil prescribed is 100 micrograms per kg daily. The patient's weight is 50 kg. So,

50 kg × 100 micrograms per kg = 5000 micrograms

The dose prescribed is 5 mg daily.

DRUG DOSES BASED ON BODY WEIGHT (CHILDREN)

This method of dosage calculation may be used but it is not a very reliable method. Young children have a high metabolic rate and may require higher doses than given by the body weight calculation. Obese children may be given too high a dose using body weight as a basis.

Calculations based on body weight of a child are carried out as shown above for adults.

DRUG DOSES BASED ON BODY SURFACE AREA (ADULTS AND CHILDREN)

Body surface area estimates are a more accurate basis on which to calculate drug doses for both adults and children, since BSA is a better indicator of metabolic processes than body weight. Body surface areas are determined by nomograms, by reference to tables or by the use of a formula.

A nomogram is a chart which relates body weight and height to body surface area. A nomogram for adults is used (Fig. 3.1). Nomograms are also available for infants and children (Haycock, Schwartz & Wisotsky 1978).

If the patient's weight and height are known (metric units are normally used), the patient's surface area can be determined as shown in Fig. 3.1. A ruler is placed across the nomogram joining the patient's height with the patient's weight. Where the 'line' crosses the central scale, the patient's BSA is given.

An alternative is to use the table in the BNF which gives a range of values for BSA from the newborn to adult males and females. These values are based on ideal body weights.

The BNF also includes a simple formula (based on BSA) for calculating doses in paediatric practice. This is based on the fact that the average BSA of a 70 kilogram adult is $1.8\,m^2$.

$$\text{Approximate dose} = \frac{\text{Surface area of patient}\,(m^2)}{1.8\,m^2} \times \text{Adult dose}$$

Thus, taking an adult dose of 250 mg for example, for a child of BSA $0.73\,m^2$,

$$\text{Approximate dose} = \frac{0.73}{1.8} \times 250\,mg$$
$$= 101.4\,mg$$

EXAMPLES OF CALCULATIONS USING BSA TO DETERMINE DOSES

Adult doses

In all cases, the BSA is obtained from the nomogram.

Example 1

Dose of epirubicin prescribed is $75\,mg/m^2$

BSA (male) is $1.8\,m^2$

Dose = Surface area of patient $(m^2) \times$ dose (mg/m^2)
$$= 1.8 \times 75$$
$$= 135\,mg$$

Example 2

Dose of idarubicin prescribed is $30\,mg/m^2$

BSA (female) is $1.6\,m^2$

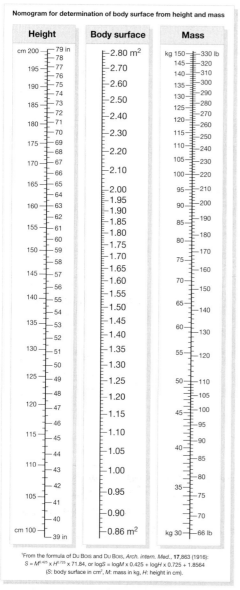

Nomogram for determination of body surface from height and mass

[Height | Body surface | Mass]

[1]From the formula of Du Bois and Du Bois, *Arch. intern. Med.*, **17**,863 (1916):
$S = M^{0.425} \times H^{0.725} \times 71.84$, or $\log S = \log M \times 0.425 + \log H \times 0.725 + 1.8564$
(S: body surface in cm², M: mass in kg, H: height in cm).

Fig. 3.1 Nomogram for adults and children

$$\text{Dose} = \text{Surface area of patient (m}^2) \times \text{dose (mg/m}^2)$$
$$= 1.6 \times 30$$
$$= 48 \, \text{mg}$$

Example 3

Dose of doxorubicin prescribed is 60 mg/m²

BSA (male) is 1.6 m²

Dose = Surface area of patient (m²) × dose (mg/m²)

     = 1.6 × 60

     = 96 mg

In most cases, the required dose should be prepared in a controlled environment in the pharmacy and presented in a ready-to-use form. If this is not the case, a further calculation may be required.

Taking the last example, doxorubicin injection is available as 2 mg in a 1 mL solution in 100 mL vials, i.e. each vial contains

    100 × 2 mg = 200 mg

The dose required according to BSA is 96 mg.

Applying the formula,

$$\frac{\text{Want (mg)}}{\text{Got (mg)}} \times \frac{\text{Volume containing}}{\text{got (mL)}} = \frac{\text{Volume containing}}{\text{required dose (mL)}} = \frac{96\,\text{mg}}{200\,\text{mg}} \times 100\,\text{mL} = 48\,\text{mL}$$

The required dose is contained in 48 mL of the injection solution. The dose for a child can also be calculated using a formula. This is a reasonably accurate guide to the dose for a child of a given surface area but should not be used in isolation from other clinically important factors.

Since most drugs are tested on young/middle-aged adults, the determination of a dose for an adult patient is generally straightforward. However, account must be taken of special factors such as renal or hepatic dysfunction; these factors may be of particular importance in the older patient.

Paediatric doses

Children and especially neonates have less well developed pathways of metabolism and excretion of drugs than adults. It follows that in determining children's doses, steps must be taken to make allowances for these differences.

The BNF gives detailed guidance on prescribing for children, including the use of body weight and body surface area. These methods are preferred to using such single factors as the age of the patient.

It is important to have an appreciation of scale in all calculations, especially when dealing with small doses for neonates and children. In order to illustrate this, a theoretical example is given below.

A dose of 500 mg (0.5 g) in a 68 kg man would be equivalent to 0.0007352% of the patient's body weight. The same dose given to a premature baby weighing 600 g would be equivalent to 0.08333% of the patient's body weight.

This demonstrates the difference in the scale of the numbers involved. When it comes to drug calculations, there is no substitute for accuracy but having an intuitive feel for numbers will provide an invaluable safety net.

When calculating for neonates or young children the doses may be very small and rounding up or down may not be appropriate as this may result in an overdose or underdose. In these cases, the exact dose must be given which may require a dilution to be made.

Dilution of solutions

There are occasions when a concentrated solution of a medicinal product must be diluted before use. In order to avoid calculation errors and possible contamination, it is preferable to use a ready-prepared solution of the required strength rather than make a dilution in the clinical area. It is recognised, however, that this may not always be possible.

Dilution of solutions for topical application may be required in a few instances (see p. 95). It is quite common for parenteral products to be diluted to a specific concentration before use (see p. 129). Some injections must be reconstituted and then diluted before use (see p. 98).

Use of calculators

Calculators should only be used to check the answer to a calculation or for making complex calculations. Nurses need to be fully competent in carrying out calculations and understand the underlying principles they are using. Over-reliance on a calculator can create a false sense of security. It should be remembered that the calculator will work on whatever figures are keyed in. If a mistake is made with a digit or the wrong sequence is entered, clearly the answer will be incorrect. Greater confidence will be reached in knowing you are able to calculate independently whether or not a calculator is available.

Drug calculations in perspective

The need to avoid errors associated with calculations is every bit as important as preventing errors in medicine administration from other causes (Downie, Mackenzie & Williams 2003). Clearly, it is essential that the patient is given the intended dose on every occasion. Those who have difficulties with calculations have a professional responsibility to address the problem by seeking help, practising repeatedly until competent and, perhaps more than anything, developing a willingness to be up front about any difficulties. There is no substitute for being observant at all times. Attention to detail is vital.

It is neither helpful nor necessary for anyone teaching this subject to create a climate of fear about drug calculations. Increasingly, medicines are being dispensed in unit doses, thus reducing the need for a calculation to be made in the clinical area. Therein, of course, lies the danger of deskilling nurses in this field, with resultant problems when a complex calculation arises. Overcoming the fears that surround calculations is as much to do with keeping the subject in perspective by providing realistic examples to practise, by not making the subject unnecessarily complicated and by instilling confidence. Those who already have mastery of the subject may be used to assist those who have not. Indeed, nurses and nursing students may learn more effectively from their peers than from more

REGULAR MEDICINES - NON-INJECTABLE

	Date Commenced	MEDICINE (Block Letters)	DOSE	ROUTE OF ADMIN	TIMES OF ADMINISTRATION								SIGNATURE	ADDITIONAL INFORMATION	DISCONTINUED		PHARMACY
					0800 hrs	1200 hrs	1400 hrs	1800 hrs	2200 hrs	OTHER TIMES					DATE	INTLS	
A																	
B																	
C																	
D																	
E																	
F																	
G																	
H																	
I																	
J																	
K																	
L																	

REGULAR MEDICINES - INJECTABLE

M																	
N																	
O																	
P																	
Q																	
R																	

ONCE ONLY MEDICINES - ALL ROUTES

Date	MEDICINE	DOSE	ROUTE OF ADMIN	TIME OF ADMIN ★	SIGNATURE	GIVEN BY	TIME IF DIFF ★

Please ✔ WHEN SPECIAL PRESCRIPTION SHEETS ARE IN USE
Fluid (Additive Medicine) Prescription Sheet
Diabetic Prescription Sheet
Oral Anticoagulant Prescription Sheet
Topical Medicines Prescription Sheet
I.V. Nutrition Sheet
Other (specify)

DRUG / MEDICINE SENSITIVITY		
Date	Medicine	Adverse Reaction

SURNAME	FORENAME	DATE OF BIRTH	UNIT NUMBER	HEIGHT / WEIGHT	HOSPITAL	WARD	CONSULTANT

Fig. 3.2 A prescription sheet.

senior staff in service and in education. Safety in the administration of medicines requires a sound understanding of how to make a calculation where it is needed. There is no place for rote learning. Calculating the dose of a medicine is an exact science; the answer is either right or it is wrong. Everyone knows which of these it must be.

NOTES ON EXAMPLES OF CALCULATIONS

The examples used to illustrate the calculation methods in this text have been chosen widely to give a cross-section of current practice. It is important to note the following:

● This is not a clinical pharmacology textbook and therefore most examples do not have supporting clinical information. Doses and routes reflect aspects of current practice but cannot cover all clinical situations that may be encountered. They should be considered as illustrative only
● It is recognised that practice does vary in different centres and that a variety of prescription forms are in use. The key point is that the prescription must contain all the relevant information and be valid according to local procedures and protocols
● Examples of labels given reflect current practice as far as this is possible within the limits of this textbook. Some abbreviations used on labels may differ from those used in the text. For example 'ml' is more commonly used than 'mL'. Occasionally non-official abbreviations may be encountered on some labels
● In order to economise on the use of space, the prescription forms used in the examples that follow (chapters 4 and 5) are necessarily incomplete. However, all the information needed to complete the calculations is shown. The full format of a prescription sheet is shown in Fig 3.2
● Labels will often be presented in various house styles. No significance should be attached to colour/design/art features, etc. In most cases, labels will give the proprietary and the approved name. All the examples have been prescribed using the approved name of the drug
● For technical reasons, some of the labels reproduced are taken from the outer pack of the product. The label reproduced gives all the necessary product information and the number of dosage units in the pack. This does not compromise the value of the exercise. It is emphasised that the label on the final container will always be the last point of reference when administering a medicine

REFERENCES

Downie G, Mackenzie J, Williams A 2003 Pharmacology and medicines management for nurses. 3rd edn. Churchill Livingstone, Edinburgh, pp 95–96.
Haycock GB, Schwartz GJ, Wisotsky DH 1978 Geometric methods for measuring body surface areas: a height-weight formula validated in infants, children and adults. Journal of Pediatrics 93(1): 62–66.
NMC 2002 Code of professional conduct. Nursing and Midwifery Council, London.

CHAPTER 4

Calculating oral and other non-injectable doses

Learning outcomes

- Be able to interpret a range of prescriptions for oral (and other non-injectable) medicines
- Be able to interpret a range of labels used for oral (and other non-injectable) medicines
- Gain practice/confidence in calculating the quantity to give the patient, using: a) reproduction prescriptions and labels b) the given information in abbreviated form (without prescription and labels)
- Be aware of the possibility of the need to dilute non-parenteral drugs prior to administration/use

---

The following pages (pp. 44–59) contain fully worked-up examples which demonstrate how to calculate doses of oral and other non-injectable drugs. Included are examples of calculations at the different levels of complexity described in Chapter 3. (Practice exercises are provided on pp. 60–94. Answers to these are given on pp. 146–148.)

A standard format is used which includes the given information, namely the prescription and the label; a few comments to provide guidance for you; the workings involved; and finally, what the patient will be given at any one time.

For various technical reasons, it has not been possible to reproduce some labels. In such cases, facsimile labels have been created. It is recognised that dispensing from bulk packs is avoided where possible. However, there may still be occasions where this is done and as a result an in house label is used.

An example of a basic calculation follows.

Example

Prescription

Regular medicines – non-injectable

Date	MEDICINE (Block Letters)	DOSE	ROUTE OF ADMIN	TIMES OF ADMINISTRATION						SIGNATURE
				0800 hrs	1200 hrs	1400 hrs	1800 hrs	2200 hrs	Other Times	
Date	SODIUM VALPROATE e/c	400 mg	ORAL	✓			✓			A Prescriber

Label (Fig. 4.1)

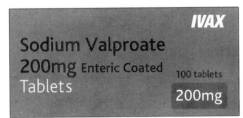

IVAX

Sodium Valproate
200mg Enteric Coated
Tablets

100 tablets

200mg

Figure 4.1   Example label.

Commentary

● This should not pose a problem for you
● Both prescription and label are expressed in milligrams

Workings
The prescribed dose is *more* than the amount contained in one tablet

$$\frac{\text{Dose required (mg)}}{\text{Strength of available tablet (mg)}}$$

$$= \frac{400\,mg}{200\,mg}$$

$$= \frac{400\,\cancel{mg}}{200\,\cancel{mg}}$$

$$= 2$$

The patient will be given:
2 tablets

After calculating the correct dose, the most suitable method of administering the medicine to the patient should be considered. Four devices are available for measuring oral and other non-injectable medicines:

● **Medicine measure (Fig. 4.2):** A standard plastic disposable container calibrated to a maximum of 30 mL from which the patient may swallow oral liquid medicines. It may also be used for conveying oral solids
● **Medicine spoon (Fig. 4.3):** A standard plastic disposable spoon which holds 5 mL of liquid. It may also be used to convey an oral solid to the patient
● **Oral syringe (Fig. 4.4):** Syringe exclusively for oral use, calibrated, complete with protective cap. For reasons of accuracy, doses for children that are less than 5 mL should be administered using an oral syringe
● **Dropper:** A glass or plastic device calibrated for use when administering small quantities of a liquid medicine

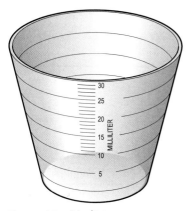

Figure 4.2 Medicine measure.

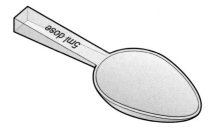

Figure 4.3 Medicine spoon.

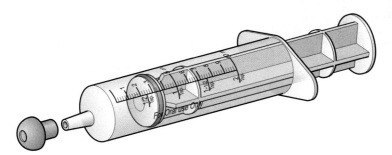

Figure 4.4 Oral syringe.

No calculation required

Example 4.1

Prescription

Regular medicines – non-injectable

Date	MEDICINE (Block Letters)	DOSE	ROUTE OF ADMIN	TIMES OF ADMINISTRATION						SIGNATURE
				0800 hrs	1200 hrs	1400 hrs	1800 hrs	2200 hrs	Other Times	
Date	ANASTROZOLE	1 mg	ORAL		✓					A. Prescriber

Label

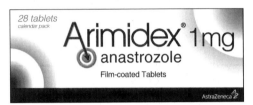

28 tablets calendar pack

Arimidex® 1mg

anastrozole

Film-coated Tablets

AstraZeneca

Commentary

● This example is completely straightforward
● No calculation is involved
● Many examples in clinical practice require no calculation
● It is essential to read the label carefully on every occasion
● The prescribed dose is the *same* as the amount contained in one tablet

The patient will be given:
1 tablet

Example 4.2

Prescription

Regular medicines – non-injectable

Date	MEDICINE (Block Letters)	DOSE	ROUTE OF ADMIN	TIMES OF ADMINISTRATION						SIGNATURE
				0800 hrs	1200 hrs	1400 hrs	1800 hrs	2200 hrs	Other Times	
Date	CHLORPROMAZINE	25 mg	ORAL	✓		✓		✓		A. Prescriber

Label

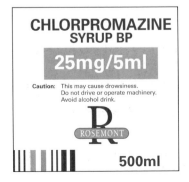

CHLORPROMAZINE
SYRUP BP

25mg/5ml

Caution: This may cause drowsiness.
Do not drive or operate machinery.
Avoid alcohol drink.

ROSEMONT

500ml

Commentary

● This is another straightforward one
● No calculation is required; it is simply a case of accurately measuring 5 mL using a medicine measure or a medicine spoon
● The prescribed dose is the *same* as the amount contained in 5 mL

The patient will be given:
5 mL of syrup

Example 4.3

Prescription

Regular medicines – non-injectable

Date	MEDICINE (Block Letters)	DOSE	ROUTE OF ADMIN	TIMES OF ADMINISTRATION							SIGNATURE
				0800 hrs	1200 hrs	1400 hrs	1800 hrs	2200 hrs	Other Times		
Date	CO-AMILOZIDE 5/50	2 tab	ORAL	✓							A. Prescriber

Label

Co-amilozide Tablets 5/50
Each tablet contains
amilozide hydrochloride 5 mg
hydrochlorothiazide 50 mg

28 tablets

Commentary

● This is a compound preparation and therefore may be prescribed in this way
● No calculation is required
● It is essential, however, that the precise strength (i.e. 5/50) is selected for administration

The patient will be given:
2 tablets

Example 4.4

Prescription

Once only medicines – all routes

Date	MEDICINE	DOSE	ROUTE OF ADMIN	TIME OF ADMIN	SIGNATURE
Date	LACTULOSE solution	15 mL	ORAL	1800 hrs	A. Prescriber

Label

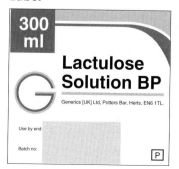

300 ml

Lactulose Solution BP

Generics [UK] Ltd, Potters Bar, Herts, EN6 1TL.

Use by end:

Batch no:

P

Commentary

● There is only one such product as lactulose solution
● The prescribed dose is written as a volume
● The volume prescribed is what the patient will be given
● The prescribed dose may be measured using a medicine measure or in the form of 3 medicine spoonfuls.

The patient will be given:
15 mL of solution

Example 4.5

Prescription

Regular medicines – non-injectable

Date	MEDICINE (Block Letters)	DOSE	ROUTE OF ADMIN	TIMES OF ADMINISTRATION						SIGNATURE
				0800 hrs	1200 hrs	1400 hrs	1800 hrs	2200 hrs	Other Times	
Date	NYSTATIN	100,000 units	ORAL	✓		✓	✓	✓		A. Prescriber

Label

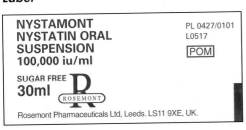

NYSTAMONT
NYSTATIN ORAL
SUSPENSION
100,000 iu/ml

PL 0427/0101
L0517
POM

SUGAR FREE
30ml ℞ ROSEMONT

Rosemont Pharmaceuticals Ltd, Leeds. LS11 9XE, UK.

Commentary

● Always note the *exact* number of zeros involved
● The prescribed dose is the *same* as the amount contained in 1 mL

The patient will be given:
1 mL of solution

Example 4.6

Prescription

Regular medicines – non-injectable

Date	MEDICINE (Block Letters)	DOSE	ROUTE OF ADMIN	TIMES OF ADMINISTRATION						SIGNATURE
				0800 hrs	1200 hrs	1400 hrs	1800 hrs	2200 hrs	Other Times	
Date	TAMSULOSIN	400 micrograms	ORAL					✓		A. Prescriber

Label

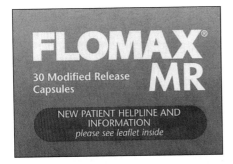

FLOMAX®
MR
30 Modified Release Capsules

NEW PATIENT HELPLINE AND INFORMATION
please see leaflet inside

Commentary

● Only the proprietary name is in evidence on this label. The BNF should be consulted to verify that Flomax® MR is a proprietary form of tamsulosin
● Always take care when dealing in micrograms
● The capsule strength does not appear on this side of the package, so all packaging must be examined. In this case the prescribed dose is the *same* as the amount contained in one capsule
● Note, product discontinued October 2005

The patient will be given:
1 capsule

LEVEL 1

Example 4.7

Prescription

Regular medicines – non-injectable

Date	MEDICINE (Block Letters)	DOSE	ROUTE OF ADMIN	TIMES OF ADMINISTRATION							SIGNATURE
				0800 hrs	1200 hrs	1400 hrs	1800 hrs	2200 hrs	Other Times		
Date	DILTIAZEM	360 mg	ORAL	✓							A. Prescriber

Label

Once Daily

Dilzem® XL 180mg
Prolonged-release Hard Capsules

diltiazem hydrochloride 180mg

for oral use
Take as directed by the physician
Do not suck or chew capsules

POM

Commentary

- A straightforward calculation
- Both prescription and label are in the same units

Workings

The prescribed dose is *more* than the amount contained in one capsule.

$$\frac{\text{Dose required}}{\text{Strength available}}$$

$$= \frac{360\,\text{mg}}{180\,\text{mg}}$$

$$= \frac{36\cancel{0}\,\cancel{\text{mg}}}{18\cancel{0}\,\cancel{\text{mg}}}$$

$$= \frac{36}{18}$$

$$= \frac{6}{3}$$

$$= 2$$

The patient will be given:
2 capsules

LEVEL 2

Example 4.8

Prescription

Regular medicines – non-injectable

Date	MEDICINE (Block Letters)	DOSE	ROUTE OF ADMIN	TIMES OF ADMINISTRATION						SIGNATURE
				0800 hrs	1200 hrs	1400 hrs	1800 hrs	2200 hrs	Other Times	
Date	DIHYDROCODEINE	30 mg	ORAL	4–6 hourly for pain						A. Prescriber

Label

150mL

**Dihydrocodeine
Oral solution
10mg/5mL**

Commentary

● A straightforward calculation
● Both prescription and label are written in milligrams and therefore no conversion is required
● A liquid preparation is involved and so the formula is advised
● Always note the strength of available product. Some are expressed per mL; some per 2 mL; and others per 5 mL
● Wherever possible, simplify fractions by dividing the figures above and below the line by the same number
● A zero cancels out another zero

Workings
The prescribed dose is *more* than the amount contained in 5 mL.

Applying the formula,

$$\frac{\text{Want}}{\text{Got}} \times \text{Volume}$$

$$= \frac{30\,\text{mg}}{10\,\text{mg}} \times 5\text{mL}$$

$$= \frac{30\,\cancel{\text{mg}}}{10\,\cancel{\text{mg}}} \times 5\text{mL}$$

$$= \frac{15}{1}\,\text{mL}$$

$$= 15\,\text{mL}$$

The patient will be given:
15 mL of oral solution

Example 4.9

Prescription

Regular medicines – non-injectable

Date	MEDICINE (Block Letters)	DOSE	ROUTE OF ADMIN	TIMES OF ADMINISTRATION							SIGNATURE
				0800 hrs	1200 hrs	1400 hrs	1800 hrs	2200 hrs	Other Times		
Date	RAMIPRIL	2.5 mg	ORAL	✓							A. Prescriber

Label

**Ramipril
Capsules
1.25mg**

28 capsules

Commentary

- Do not be alarmed by decimal points
- Both prescription and label are written in milligrams
- Remember when moving a decimal point, to do so the *same* number of places in the *same* direction above *and* below the line

Workings

The prescribed dose is *more* than the amount contained in one capsule.

$$= \frac{\text{Dose required}}{\text{Strength available}}$$

$$= \frac{2.5\,\text{mg}}{1.25\,\text{mg}}$$

$$= \frac{2.50\,\text{mg}}{1.25\,\text{mg}}$$

$$= \frac{250}{125}$$

$$= 2$$

The patient will be given:

2 capsules

Example 4.10

Prescription

Once only medicines – all routes

Date	MEDICINE	DOSE	ROUTE OF ADMIN	TIME OF ADMIN	SIGNATURE
Date	PARACETAMOL	1g	ORAL	0930 hrs	A. Prescriber

Label

**Paracetamol
Tablets
500mg**

32 Tablets

Commentary

The prescription and label are written in different units and therefore a conversion is required

Workings

The prescribed dose is *more* than the amount contained in one tablet.

First, 1 g must be converted to milligrams: 1g = 1000 mg

$$= \frac{\text{Dose required}}{\text{Strength available}}$$

$$= \frac{1000\,\text{mg}}{500\,\text{mg}}$$

$$= \frac{1000\,\text{mg}}{500\,\text{mg}}$$

$$= \frac{10^2}{5_1}$$

$$= 2$$

The patient will be given:
2 tablets

Example 4.11

Prescription

Regular medicines – non-injectable

Date	MEDICINE (Block Letters)	DOSE	ROUTE OF ADMIN	TIMES OF ADMINISTRATION						SIGNATURE
				0800 hrs	1200 hrs	1400 hrs	1800 hrs	2200 hrs	Other Times	
Date	BACLOFEN	5 mg	ORAL	✓		✓		✓	for 3 days	A. Prescriber
Date	BACLOFEN	2.5 mg	ORAL	✓		✓		✓	for 7 days	A. Prescriber

Label

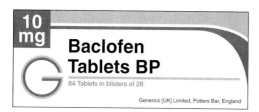

10 mg

Baclofen Tablets BP

84 Tablets in blisters of 28

Generics [UK] Limited, Potters Bar, England

Commentary

● A separate calculation is required for each prescription

Workings

Each of the prescribed doses is *less* than the amount contained in one tablet.

1. First prescription

$$\frac{\text{Dose required}}{\text{Strength available}}$$

$$= \frac{5\,\text{mg}}{10\,\text{mg}}$$

$$= \frac{\overset{1}{\cancel{5}}\,\text{mg}}{\underset{2}{\cancel{10}}\,\text{mg}}$$

$$= \frac{1}{2}$$

2. Second prescription

$$\frac{\text{Dose required}}{\text{Strength available}}$$

$$= \frac{2.5\,\text{mg}}{10\,\text{mg}}$$

$$= \frac{2.5\,\cancel{\text{mg}}}{10.0\,\cancel{\text{mg}}}$$

$$= \frac{25}{100}$$

$$= \frac{1}{4}$$

The patient will be given:

1. Half a 10 mg tablet

2. Quarter of a 10 mg tablet

LEVEL 3

Example 4.12

Prescription

Regular medicines – non-injectable

Date	MEDICINE (Block Letters)	DOSE	ROUTE OF ADMIN	TIMES OF ADMINISTRATION							SIGNATURE
				0800 hrs	1200 hrs	1400 hrs	1800 hrs	2200 hrs	Other Times		
Date	ALFACALCIDOL	1 microgram	ORAL	✓							A. Prescriber

Label

One-Alpha®
Capsules
0.25 microgram
alfacalcidol

30 capsules

Commentary

● The prescription and the label are in different units and therefore a conversion is required
● We are working here with very low strengths and so great care must be taken

Workings

The prescribed dose is *more* than the amount in one capsule.

Converting 1 microgram to nanograms,

1000 nanograms = 1 microgram

$$\frac{\text{Dose required}}{\text{Strength available}}$$

$$= \frac{1000 \text{ nanograms}}{250 \text{ nanograms}}$$

$$= \frac{\overset{4}{\cancel{1000}} \text{ nanograms}}{\underset{1}{\cancel{250}} \text{ nanograms}}$$

$$= 4$$

The patient will be given:
4 capsules

Example 4.13

Prescription

Regular medicines – non-injectable

Date	MEDICINE (Block Letters)	DOSE	ROUTE OF ADMIN	TIMES OF ADMINISTRATION							SIGNATURE
				0800 hrs	1200 hrs	1400 hrs	1800 hrs	2200 hrs	Other Times		
Date	AZATHIOPRINE	1.5 mg/kg	ORAL		✓						A. Prescriber

Label

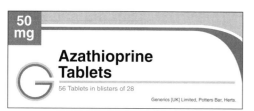

Azathioprine Tablets
56 Tablets in blisters of 28

Generics [UK] Limited, Potters Bar, Herts.

Commentary

● Let's assume the patient weighs 52 kg
● Depending on the patient's weight, the calculation may result in an odd figure and therefore the patient will be given the nearest approximate amount

Workings

Multiply prescribed dose by patient's weight, i.e.

$$1.5\,mg \times 52 = 78\,mg$$

$$\frac{\text{Dose required}}{\text{Strength available}}$$

$$= \frac{78\,mg}{50\,mg}$$

$$= \frac{78\,\cancel{mg}}{50\,\cancel{mg}}$$

$$= \text{approx.}\ 1\frac{1}{2}$$

The patient will be given:

$1\frac{1}{2}$ tablets

Example 4.14

Prescription

Regular medicines – non-injectable

Date	MEDICINE (Block Letters)	DOSE	ROUTE OF ADMIN	TIMES OF ADMINISTRATION							SIGNATURE
				0800 hrs	1200 hrs	1400 hrs	1800 hrs	2200 hrs	Other Times		
Date	DIGOXIN elixir	175 micrograms	ORAL	✓							A. Prescriber

Label

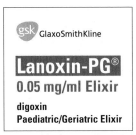

Commentary

● At a glance, you may not be able to judge whether the prescribed dose is *more* or *less* than the amount contained in 1 mL of elixir

Workings

Change 0.05 mg to micrograms,

∴ multiply 0.05 by 1000,

i.e. move decimal point 3 places to the right,

$$0.0\widetilde{50}$$

$$= 0050.$$

$$= 50$$

∴ 0.05 mg = 50 micrograms

Applying the formula,

$$\frac{\text{Want}}{\text{Got}} \times \text{Volume}$$

$$= \frac{175 \text{ micrograms}}{50 \text{ micrograms}} \times 1\text{mL}$$

$$= \frac{\overset{7}{\cancel{175}} \text{ micrograms}}{\underset{2}{\cancel{50}} \text{ micrograms}} \times 1\text{mL}$$

$$= \frac{7}{2} \text{mL}$$

$$= 3.5 \text{mL}$$

The patient will be given:
3.5 mL elixir

Example 4.15

Prescription

Regular medicines – non-injectable

Date	MEDICINE (Block Letters)	DOSE	ROUTE OF ADMIN	TIMES OF ADMINISTRATION						SIGNATURE
				0800 hrs	1200 hrs	1400 hrs	1800 hrs	2200 hrs	Other Times	
Date	LITHIUM CITRATE	10.8 mmol	ORAL	✓						A. Prescriber

Label

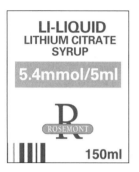

LI-LIQUID
LITHIUM CITRATE
SYRUP

5.4mmol/5ml

ROSEMONT

150ml

Commentary

- Doses of oral drugs are seldom expressed in millimoles
- Here, both prescription and label are expressed in millimoles and therefore there is no difference to working out the calculation

Workings

The prescribed dose is *more* than the amount contained in 5 mL of oral solution.

Using the formula,

$$\frac{\text{Want}}{\text{Got}} \times \text{Volume}$$

$$= \frac{10.8 \text{ mmol}}{5.4 \text{ mmol}} \times 5 \text{ mL}$$

$$= \frac{10.8 \text{ mmol}}{5.4 \text{ mmol}} \times 5 \text{ mL}$$

$$= \frac{108}{54} \times 5 \text{ mL}$$

$$= \frac{^2\cancel{108}}{\cancel{54}_1} \times 5 \text{ mL}$$

$$= 10 \text{ mL}$$

The patient will be given:
10 mL of syrup

Example 4.16

Prescription

Regular medicines – non-injectable

Date	MEDICINE (Block Letters)	DOSE	ROUTE OF ADMIN	0800 hrs	1200 hrs	1400 hrs	1800 hrs	2200 hrs	Other Times	SIGNATURE
				TIMES OF ADMINISTRATION						
Date	MYCOPHENOLATE MOFETIL	600 mg/m²	ORAL	✓			✓			A. Prescriber

Label

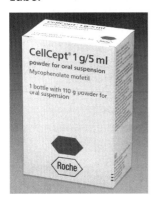

CellCept® 1 g/5 ml
powder for oral suspension
Mycophenolate mofetil

1 bottle with 110 g powder for
oral suspension

Roche

Commentary

● Let us say the patient's BSA is 1.6 m²

Workings

First, convert 1 g to milligrams

$1 g = 1000 mg$

The prescribed dose is multiplied by the patient's BSA, i.e.

$600 mg \times 1.6 m^2 = 960 mg$

Applying the formula,

$$\frac{Want}{Got} \times Volume$$

$$= \frac{960 mg}{1000 mg} \times 5 mL$$

$$= \frac{960 \, \cancel{mg}}{1000 \, \cancel{mg}} \times 5 mL$$

$$= \frac{96}{\cancel{100}_{20}} \times \cancel{5}^{1} mL$$

$$= \frac{96}{20} mL$$

$$= \frac{24}{5} mL$$

$$= 4 \frac{4}{5} mL$$

$$= 4.8 mL$$

The patient will be given:
4.8 mL of suspension

Example 4.17

Prescription

Once only medicines – all routes

Date	MEDICINE	DOSE	ROUTE OF ADMIN	TIME OF ADMIN	SIGNATURE
Date	BERACTANT	100 mg/kg	ET tube	0800 hrs	A. Prescriber

Label

> **Beractant Suspension 25mg/mL**
>
> 8mL vial

Commentary

- This drug is administered by a special route, i.e. via endotracheal tube
- The patient is a baby weighing 1.8 kg

Workings

$$\text{Dose} = 100 \times 1.8\,\text{mg}$$
$$= 180\,\text{mg}$$

The prescribed dose is *more* than the amount contained in 1 mL of suspension.

Applying the formula,

$$\frac{\text{Want}}{\text{Got}} \times \text{Volume}$$

$$= \frac{180\,\text{mg}}{25\,\text{mg}} \times 1\,\text{mL}$$

$$= \frac{36}{5}\,\text{mL}$$

$$= 7\frac{1}{5}\,\text{mL}$$

$$= 7.2\,\text{mL}$$

The patient will be given:
7.2 mL suspension via ET tube

Practice exercises (answers on pp. 146–148)

LEVEL 1

Exercise 4.1

Prescription

Regular medicines – non-injectable

Date	MEDICINE (Block Letters)	DOSE	ROUTE OF ADMIN	TIMES OF ADMINISTRATION						SIGNATURE
				0800 hrs	1200 hrs	1400 hrs	1800 hrs	2200 hrs	Other Times	
Date	BISACODYL	10 mg	ORAL					✓		A. Prescriber

Label

Bisacodyl Tablets 5mg

10 Tablets

Exercise 4.2

Prescription

Regular medicines – non-injectable

Date	MEDICINE (Block Letters)	DOSE	ROUTE OF ADMIN	TIMES OF ADMINISTRATION						SIGNATURE
				0800 hrs	1200 hrs	1400 hrs	1800 hrs	2200 hrs	Other Times	
Date	DOXEPIN	40 mg	ORAL		✓					A. Prescriber

Label

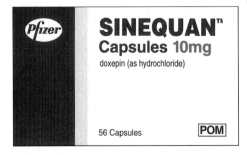

SINEQUAN™
Capsules 10mg
doxepin (as hydrochloride)

56 Capsules   **POM**

Exercise 4.3

Prescription

Regular medicines – non-injectable

Date	MEDICINE (Block Letters)	DOSE	ROUTE OF ADMIN	TIMES OF ADMINISTRATION						SIGNATURE
				0800 hrs	1200 hrs	1400 hrs	1800 hrs	2200 hrs	Other Times	
Date	ASPIRIN dispersible	150 mg	ORAL	✓						A. Prescriber

Label

⊘X PHARMACEUTICALS
Dispersible Aspirin Tablets BP 75mg
28 tablets

Exercise 4.4

Prescription

Regular medicines – non-injectable

Date	MEDICINE (Block Letters)	DOSE	ROUTE OF ADMIN	TIMES OF ADMINISTRATION						SIGNATURE
				0800 hrs	1200 hrs	1400 hrs	1800 hrs	2200 hrs	Other Times	
Date	DIAZEPAM	3 mg	ORAL	✓		✓		✓		A. Prescriber

Label

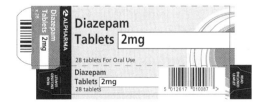

Commentary

- Sometimes there is no alternative but to divide a tablet
- A tablet splitter should be used for accuracy

Exercise 4.5

Prescription

Regular medicines – non-injectable

Date	MEDICINE (Block Letters)	DOSE	ROUTE OF ADMIN	TIMES OF ADMINISTRATION						SIGNATURE
				0800 hrs	1200 hrs	1400 hrs	1800 hrs	2200 hrs	Other Times	
Date	MIRTAZAPINE	45 mg	ORAL					✓		A. Prescriber

Label

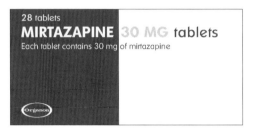

28 tablets
MIRTAZAPINE 30 MG tablets
Each tablet contains 30 mg of mirtazapine

Organon

Exercise 4.6

Prescription

Regular medicines – non-injectable

Date	MEDICINE (Block Letters)	DOSE	ROUTE OF ADMIN	TIMES OF ADMINISTRATION						SIGNATURE
				0800 hrs	1200 hrs	1400 hrs	1800 hrs	2200 hrs	Other Times	
Date	LIOTHYRONINE	10 micrograms	ORAL	✓						A. Prescriber

Label

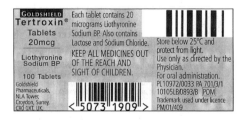

GOLDSHIELD
Tertroxin®
Tablets
20mcg

Liothyronine
Sodium BP

100 Tablets
Goldshield
Pharmaceuticals,
NLA Tower,
Croydon, Surrey,
CR0 0XT. UK.

Each tablet contains 20 micrograms Liothyronine Sodium BP. Also contains Lactose and Sodium Chloride.

KEEP ALL MEDICINES OUT OF THE REACH AND SIGHT OF CHILDREN.

Store below 25°C and protect from light. Use only as directed by the Physician. For oral administration.
PL10972/0033 PA 701/3/1
10105LB/0893/B POM
Trademark used under licence
PM/01/409

5073 1909

Commentary

● Take great care when working in micrograms

Exercise 4.7

Prescription

Regular medicines – non-injectable

Date	MEDICINE (Block Letters)	DOSE	ROUTE OF ADMIN	TIMES OF ADMINISTRATION							SIGNATURE
				0800 hrs	1200 hrs	1400 hrs	1800 hrs	2200 hrs	Other Times		
Date	PREDNISOLONE E/C	60 mg	ORAL	✓							A. Prescriber

Label

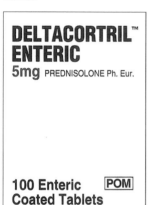

DELTACORTRIL™ ENTERIC
5mg PREDNISOLONE Ph. Eur.

100 Enteric Coated Tablets | POM |

Commentary

- It is not common to have to give patients as many tablets to reach the dose as in this example
- *Always* get someone else to check, if you are in any doubt about what to give the patient

Exercise 4.8

Prescription

Regular medicines – non-injectable

Date	MEDICINE (Block Letters)	DOSE	ROUTE OF ADMIN	TIMES OF ADMINISTRATION							SIGNATURE
				0800 hrs	1200 hrs	1400 hrs	1800 hrs	2200 hrs	Other Times		
Date	WARFARIN	6 mg	ORAL				✓				A. Prescriber

Label

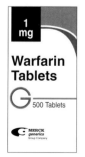

1 mg
Warfarin Tablets
500 Tablets
MERCK generics Group Company

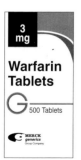

3 mg
Warfarin Tablets
500 Tablets
MERCK generics Group Company

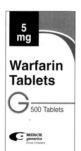

5 mg
Warfarin Tablets
500 Tablets
MERCK generics Group Company

Commentary

- There are three strengths of warfarin available
- You have to select a suitable combination of strengths that will provide the prescribed dose
- Your calculation should result in the minimum number of tablets the patient has to take
- As a rule of thumb, it is probably best always to start with the highest strength possible and then add what is required to reach the prescribed dose

Exercise 4.9

Prescription

Regular medicines – non-injectable

Date	MEDICINE (Block Letters)	DOSE	ROUTE OF ADMIN	TIMES OF ADMINISTRATION							SIGNATURE
				0800 hrs	1200 hrs	1400 hrs	1800 hrs	2200 hrs	Other Times		
Date	PHENYTOIN	300 mg	ORAL		✓						A. Prescriber

Label

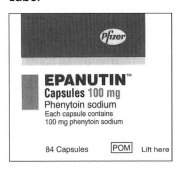

Exercise 4.10

Prescription

Regular medicines – non-injectable

Date	MEDICINE (Block Letters)	DOSE	ROUTE OF ADMIN	TIMES OF ADMINISTRATION							SIGNATURE
				0800 hrs	1200 hrs	1400 hrs	1800 hrs	2200 hrs	Other Times		
Date	RANITIDINE	300 mg	ORAL					✓			A. Prescriber

Label

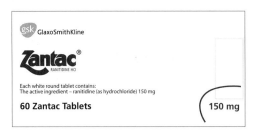

Exercise 4.11

Prescription

Regular medicines – non-injectable

Date	MEDICINE (Block Letters)	DOSE	ROUTE OF ADMIN	TIMES OF ADMINISTRATION							SIGNATURE
				0800 hrs	1200 hrs	1400 hrs	1800 hrs	2200 hrs	Other Times		
Date	BISOPROLOL	20 mg	ORAL	✓							A. Prescriber

Label

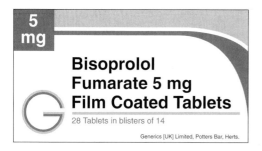

Exercise 4.12

Prescription

Regular medicines – non-injectable

Date	MEDICINE (Block Letters)	DOSE	ROUTE OF ADMIN	TIMES OF ADMINISTRATION							SIGNATURE
				0800 hrs	1200 hrs	1400 hrs	1800 hrs	2200 hrs	Other Times		
Date	BACLOFEN	5 mg	ORAL	✓		✓	✓				A. Prescriber

Label

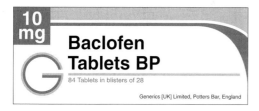

Exercise 4.13

Prescription

Regular medicines – non-injectable

Date	MEDICINE (Block Letters)	DOSE	ROUTE OF ADMIN	TIMES OF ADMINISTRATION							SIGNATURE
				0800 hrs	1200 hrs	1400 hrs	1800 hrs	2200 hrs	Other Times		
Date	ATENOLOL	75 mg	ORAL	✓							A. Prescriber

Label

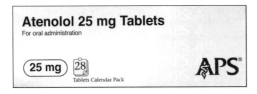

Atenolol 25 mg Tablets
For oral administration

25 mg 28 Tablets Calendar Pack APS®

Exercise 4.14

Prescription

Regular medicines – non-injectable

Date	MEDICINE (Block Letters)	DOSE	ROUTE OF ADMIN	TIMES OF ADMINISTRATION							SIGNATURE
				0800 hrs	1200 hrs	1400 hrs	1800 hrs	2200 hrs	Other Times		
Date	BETAHISTINE	16 mg	ORAL with food	✓	✓		✓				A. Prescriber

Label

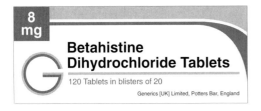

8 mg

Betahistine Dihydrochloride Tablets

120 Tablets in blisters of 20

Generics [UK] Limited, Potters Bar, England

Exercise 4.15

Prescription

Regular medicines – non-injectable

Date	MEDICINE (Block Letters)	DOSE	ROUTE OF ADMIN	TIMES OF ADMINISTRATION							SIGNATURE
				0800 hrs	1200 hrs	1400 hrs	1800 hrs	2200 hrs	Other Times		
Date	CODEINE PHOSPHATE	60 mg	ORAL	✓	✓		✓	✓			A. Prescriber

Label

**Codeine phosphate
Tablets
30mg**

30 tablets

Exercise 4.16

Prescription

Regular medicines – non-injectable

Date	MEDICINE (Block Letters)	DOSE	ROUTE OF ADMIN	TIMES OF ADMINISTRATION							SIGNATURE
				0800 hrs	1200 hrs	1400 hrs	1800 hrs	2200 hrs	Other Times		
Date	ALLOPURINOL	200 mg	ORAL	✓		✓	✓				A. Prescriber

Label

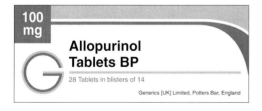

**100
mg**

**Allopurinol
Tablets BP**

28 Tablets in blisters of 14

Generics [UK] Limited, Potters Bar, England

Exercise 4.17

Prescription

Regular medicines – non-injectable

Date	MEDICINE (Block Letters)	DOSE	ROUTE OF ADMIN	TIMES OF ADMINISTRATION						SIGNATURE
				0800 hrs	1200 hrs	1400 hrs	1800 hrs	2200 hrs	Other Times	
Date	AMLODIPINE	10 mg	ORAL	✓						A. Prescriber

Label

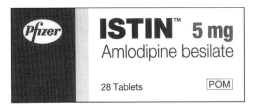

ISTIN™ 5 mg
Amlodipine besilate

Pfizer

28 Tablets   POM

Exercise 4.18

Prescription

Regular medicines – non-injectable

Date	MEDICINE (Block Letters)	DOSE	ROUTE OF ADMIN	TIMES OF ADMINISTRATION						SIGNATURE
				0800 hrs	1200 hrs	1400 hrs	1800 hrs	2200 hrs	Other Times	
Date	SOLUBLE ASPIRIN	900 mg	ORAL	6 hourly if required for pain						A. Prescriber

Label

**Soluble aspirin
Tablets
300mg**

100 Tablets

Exercise 4.19

Prescription

Regular medicines – non-injectable

Date	MEDICINE (Block Letters)	DOSE	ROUTE OF ADMIN	0800 hrs	1200 hrs	1400 hrs	1800 hrs	2200 hrs	Other Times		SIGNATURE
				TIMES OF ADMINISTRATION							
Date	FUROSEMIDE	30 mg	ORAL	✓							A. Prescriber

Label

**Furosemide
Tablets
20mg**

28 Tablets

LEVEL II

Exercise 4.20

Prescription

Once only medicines – all routes

Date	MEDICINE	DOSE	ROUTE OF ADMIN	TIME OF ADMIN	SIGNATURE
Date	LOPERAMIDE	4 mg	ORAL	1130 hrs	A. Prescriber

Label

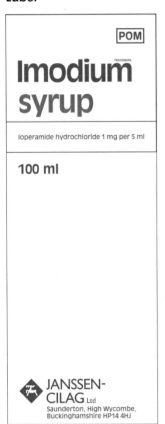

POM

Imodium TRADEMARK
syrup

loperamide hydrochloride 1 mg per 5 ml

100 ml

JANSSEN-
CILAG Ltd
Saunderton, High Wycombe,
Buckinghamshire HP14 4HJ

Exercise 4.21

Prescription

Regular medicines – non-injectable

Date	MEDICINE (Block Letters)	DOSE	ROUTE OF ADMIN	TIMES OF ADMINISTRATION							SIGNATURE
				0800 hrs	1200 hrs	1400 hrs	1800 hrs	2200 hrs	Other Times		
Date	ERYTHROMYCIN	250 mg	ORAL	✓		✓		✓			A. Prescriber

Label

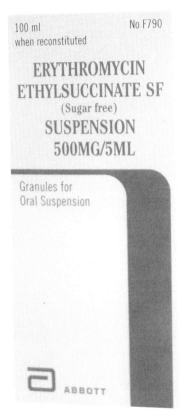

100 ml
when reconstituted

No F790

ERYTHROMYCIN ETHYLSUCCINATE SF
(Sugar free)
**SUSPENSION
500MG/5ML**

Granules for
Oral Suspension

ABBOTT

Exercise 4.22

Prescription

Regular medicines – non-injectable

Date	MEDICINE (Block Letters)	DOSE	ROUTE OF ADMIN	TIMES OF ADMINISTRATION							SIGNATURE
				0800 hrs	1200 hrs	1400 hrs	1800 hrs	2200 hrs	Other Times		
Date	PROCYCLIDINE	2.5 mg	ORAL	✓		✓		✓			A. Prescriber

Label

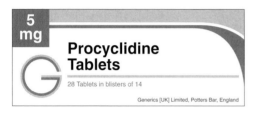

5 mg

Procyclidine Tablets

28 Tablets in blisters of 14

Generics [UK] Limited, Potters Bar, England

Exercise 4.23

Prescription

Regular medicines – non-injectable

Date	MEDICINE (Block Letters)	DOSE	ROUTE OF ADMIN	TIMES OF ADMINISTRATION							SIGNATURE
				0800 hrs	1200 hrs	1400 hrs	1800 hrs	2200 hrs	Other Times		
Date	BENDROFLUME-THIAZIDE	5 mg	ORAL	✓							A. Prescriber

Label

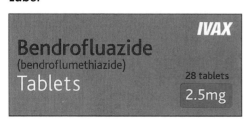

IVAX

Bendrofluazide
(bendroflumethiazide)
Tablets

28 tablets

2.5mg

Commentary

● Note change of proprietary name

Exercise 4.24

Prescription

Regular medicines – non-injectable

Date	MEDICINE (Block Letters)	DOSE	ROUTE OF ADMIN	TIMES OF ADMINISTRATION						SIGNATURE
				0800 hrs	1200 hrs	1400 hrs	1800 hrs	2200 hrs	Other Times	
Date	SODIUM VALPROATE	300 mg	ORAL	✓			✓			A. Prescriber

Label

100mL

**Sodium valproate
Oral solution
200mg/5mL**

Exercise 4.25

Prescription

Regular medicines – non-injectable

Date	MEDICINE (Block Letters)	DOSE	ROUTE OF ADMIN	TIMES OF ADMINISTRATION						SIGNATURE
				0800 hrs	1200 hrs	1400 hrs	1800 hrs	2200 hrs	Other Times	
Date	HALOPERIDOL	1 mg	ORAL	✓			✓			A. Prescriber

Label

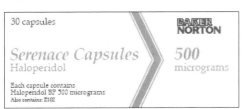

30 capsules

BAKER NORTON

Serenace Capsules
Haloperidol

500 micrograms

Each capsule contains
Haloperidol BP 500 micrograms
Also contains: E102

Exercise 4.26

Prescription

Regular medicines – non-injectable

Date	MEDICINE (Block Letters)	DOSE	ROUTE OF ADMIN	TIMES OF ADMINISTRATION							SIGNATURE
				0800 hrs	1200 hrs	1400 hrs	1800 hrs	2200 hrs	Other Times		
Date	RISPERIDONE	500 micrograms	ORAL	✓			✓				A. Prescriber

Label

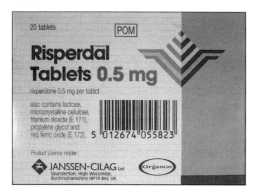

Exercise 4.27

Prescription

Regular medicines – non-injectable

Date	MEDICINE (Block Letters)	DOSE	ROUTE OF ADMIN	TIMES OF ADMINISTRATION							SIGNATURE
				0800 hrs	1200 hrs	1400 hrs	1800 hrs	2200 hrs	Other Times		
Date	AMOXICILLIN	500 mg	ORAL	✓	✓		✓	✓			A. Prescriber

Label

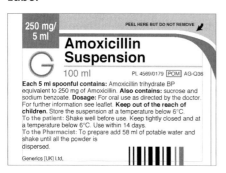

Exercise 4.28

Prescription

Once only medicines – all routes

Date	MEDICINE	DOSE	ROUTE OF ADMIN	TIME OF ADMIN	SIGNATURE
Date	COLCHICINE	1 mg	ORAL	1130 hrs	A. Prescriber

Label

**Colchicine
Tablets
500 micrograms**

28 tablets

Exercise 4.29

Prescription

Regular medicines – non-injectable

Date	MEDICINE (Block Letters)	DOSE	ROUTE OF ADMIN	TIMES OF ADMINISTRATION						SIGNATURE
				0800 hrs	1200 hrs	1400 hrs	1800 hrs	2200 hrs	Other Times	
Date	AZITHROMYCIN	300 mg	ORAL		✓					A. Prescriber

Label

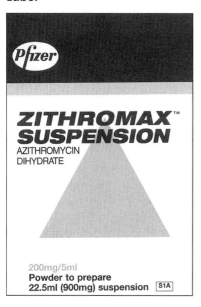

Exercise 4.30

Prescription

Regular medicines – non-injectable

Date	MEDICINE (Block Letters)	DOSE	ROUTE OF ADMIN	TIMES OF ADMINISTRATION						SIGNATURE
				0800 hrs	1200 hrs	1400 hrs	1800 hrs	2200 hrs	Other Times	
Date	FERROUS GLYCINE SULPHATE ELEMENTAL IRON	30 mg	ORAL	✓	✓		✓			A. Prescriber

Label

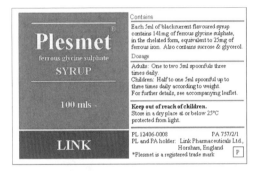

Exercise 4.31

Prescription

Regular medicines – non-injectable

Date	MEDICINE (Block Letters)	DOSE	ROUTE OF ADMIN	TIMES OF ADMINISTRATION						SIGNATURE
				0800 hrs	1200 hrs	1400 hrs	1800 hrs	2200 hrs	Other Times	
Date	SALBUTAMOL	200 micrograms	INHAL	✓	✓		✓			A. Prescriber

Label

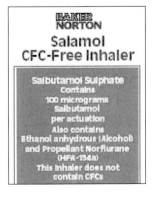

Exercise 4.32

Prescription

Regular medicines – non-injectable

Date	MEDICINE (Block Letters)	DOSE	ROUTE OF ADMIN	TIMES OF ADMINISTRATION							SIGNATURE
				0800 hrs	1200 hrs	1400 hrs	1800 hrs	2200 hrs	Other Times	
Date	PROMAZINE	200 mg	ORAL	✓	✓		✓	✓		A. Prescriber

Label

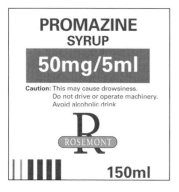

PROMAZINE
SYRUP
50mg/5ml

Caution: This may cause drowsiness.
Do not drive or operate machinery.
Avoid alcoholic drink

℞
ROSEMONT

150ml

Exercise 4.33

Prescription

Regular medicines – non-injectable

Date	MEDICINE (Block Letters)	DOSE	ROUTE OF ADMIN	TIMES OF ADMINISTRATION							SIGNATURE
				0800 hrs	1200 hrs	1400 hrs	1800 hrs	2200 hrs	Other Times	
Date	SODIUM PICOSULFATE	10 mg	ORAL					✓		A. Prescriber

Label

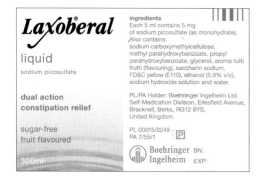

Laxoberal®

liquid
sodium picosulfate

dual action
constipation relief

sugar-free
fruit flavoured

300ml

ingredients
Each 5 ml contains 5 mg
of sodium picosulfate (as monohydrate).
Also contains:
sodium carboxymethylcellulose,
methyl parahydroxybenzoate, propyl
parahydroxybenzoate, glycerol, aroma tutti
frutti (flavouring), saccharin sodium,
FD&C yellow (E110), ethanol (5.9% v/v),
sodium hydroxide solution and water.

PL/PA Holder: Boehringer Ingelheim Ltd.
Self-Medication Division, Ellesfield Avenue,
Bracknell, Berks, RG12 8YS,
United Kingdom.

PL 00015/0249
PA 7/55/1 Ⓟ

Boehringer BN:
Ingelheim EXP:

Exercise 4.34

Prescription

Regular medicines – non-injectable

Date	MEDICINE (Block Letters)	DOSE	ROUTE OF ADMIN	TIMES OF ADMINISTRATION						SIGNATURE
				0800 hrs	1200 hrs	1400 hrs	1800 hrs	2200 hrs	Other Times	
Date	CHLORPROMAZINE	75 mg	ORAL					✓		A. Prescriber

Label

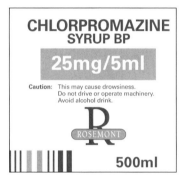

CHLORPROMAZINE
SYRUP BP
25mg/5ml

Caution: This may cause drowsiness. Do not drive or operate machinery. Avoid alcohol drink.

ROSEMONT

500ml

Exercise 4.35

Prescription

Regular medicines – non-injectable

Date	MEDICINE (Block Letters)	DOSE	ROUTE OF ADMIN	TIMES OF ADMINISTRATION						SIGNATURE
				0800 hrs	1200 hrs	1400 hrs	1800 hrs	2200 hrs	Other Times	
Date	DIHYDROCODEINE	30 mg	ORAL	Every 4–6 hours for pain						A. Prescriber

Label

150mL

Dihydrocodeine Elixir 10mg/5mL

Exercise 4.36

Prescription

Regular medicines – non-injectable

Date	MEDICINE (Block Letters)	DOSE	ROUTE OF ADMIN	TIMES OF ADMINISTRATION						SIGNATURE
				0800 hrs	1200 hrs	1400 hrs	1800 hrs	2200 hrs	Other Times	
Date	MORPHINE	15 mg	ORAL	Every 4–6 hours for pain						A. Prescriber

Label

Oramorph® Concentrated Oral Solution	Warning. May cause drowsiness. If affected do not drive or operate machinery. Avoid alcoholic drink.
morphine sulphate	Keep out of the sight and reach of children
	To be taken as directed by the prescriber
20 mg/ml	See enclosed leaflet for further information
120 ml	Do not store above 25°C. Protect from light.
bottle with dropper	This product also contains disodium edetate, sodium benzoate, citric acid, amaranth and purified water.
	Discard 120 days after opening
Each 1 ml contains Morphine Sulphate 20 mg	Date opened / /
This bottle contains a total of 2400 mg of morphine sulphate	PL 0015/0125 CD POM
	PA7/44/2
	HOSPITAL DIVISION Boehringer Ingelheim Ltd., Bracknell, Berkshire, RG12 8YS United Kingdom

Exercise 4.37

Prescription

Regular medicines – non-injectable

Date	MEDICINE (Block Letters)	DOSE	ROUTE OF ADMIN	TIMES OF ADMINISTRATION						SIGNATURE
				0800 hrs	1200 hrs	1400 hrs	1800 hrs	2200 hrs	Other Times	
Date	CIPROFLOXACIN	750 mg	ORAL	✓			✓			A. Prescriber

Label

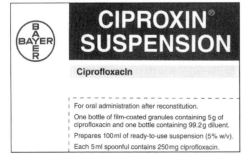

CIPROXIN® SUSPENSION

Ciprofloxacin

For oral administration after reconstitution.

One bottle of film-coated granules containing 5 g of ciprofloxacin and one bottle containing 99.2 g diluent.

Prepares 100 ml of ready-to-use suspension (5% w/v).

Each 5 ml spoonful contains 250 mg ciprofloxacin.

Exercise 4.38

Prescription

Regular medicines – non-injectable

Date	MEDICINE (Block Letters)	DOSE	ROUTE OF ADMIN	TIMES OF ADMINISTRATION							SIGNATURE
				0800 hrs	1200 hrs	1400 hrs	1800 hrs	2200 hrs	Other Times		
Date	FLUPENTIXOL	500 micrograms	ORAL	✓							A. Prescriber

Label

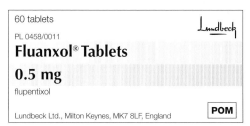

60 tablets

PL 0458/0011

Fluanxol® Tablets

0.5 mg

flupentixol

Lundbeck Ltd., Milton Keynes, MK7 8LF, England

POM

Exercise 4.39

Prescription

Regular medicines – non-injectable

Date	MEDICINE (Block Letters)	DOSE	ROUTE OF ADMIN	TIMES OF ADMINISTRATION						SIGNATURE
				0800 hrs	1200 hrs	1400 hrs	1800 hrs	2200 hrs	Other Times	
Date	LAMIVUDINE	80 mg	ORAL		✓					A. Prescriber

Label

Zeffix® 5 mg/ml
oral solution
Lamivudine

Bottle contents:
240 ml oral solution
containing
5 mg/ml lamivudine

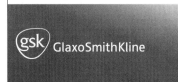 GlaxoSmithKline

Exercise 4.40

Prescription

Regular medicines – non-injectable

Date	MEDICINE (Block Letters)	DOSE	ROUTE OF ADMIN	TIMES OF ADMINISTRATION						SIGNATURE
				0800 hrs	1200 hrs	1400 hrs	1800 hrs	2200 hrs	Other Times	
Date	CHLORPHENAMINE	1 mg	ORAL	Every 4–6 hours if required for itch						A. Prescriber

Label

```
150mL

Chlorphenamine
Oral solution
2mg/5mL
```

Exercise 4.41

Prescription

Regular medicines – non-injectable

Date	MEDICINE (Block Letters)	DOSE	ROUTE OF ADMIN	TIMES OF ADMINISTRATION						SIGNATURE
				0800 hrs	1200 hrs	1400 hrs	1800 hrs	2200 hrs	Other Times	
Date	PARACETAMOL	375 mg	ORAL	Every 4–6 hours as required for pain						A. Prescriber

Label

```
100mL

Paracetamol
Oral suspension
250mg/5mL
```

Exercise 4.42

Prescription

Regular medicines – non-injectable

Date	MEDICINE (Block Letters)	DOSE	ROUTE OF ADMIN	TIMES OF ADMINISTRATION						SIGNATURE
				0800 hrs	1200 hrs	1400 hrs	1800 hrs	2200 hrs	Other Times	
Date	SULFASALAZINE	1.5 g	ORAL	✓	✓		✓	✓		A. Prescriber

Label

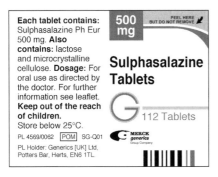

Each tablet contains: Sulphasalazine Ph Eur 500 mg. **Also contains:** lactose and microcrystalline cellulose. **Dosage:** For oral use as directed by the doctor. For further information see leaflet. **Keep out of the reach of children.** Store below 25°C.

PL 4569/0062 [POM] SG-Q01

PL Holder: Generics [UK] Ltd, Potters Bar, Herts, EN6 1TL.

500 mg PEEL HERE BUT DO NOT REMOVE

Sulphalazine Tablets

112 Tablets

MERCK generics Group Company

Exercise 4.43

Prescription

Regular medicines – non-injectable

Date	MEDICINE (Block Letters)	DOSE	ROUTE OF ADMIN	TIMES OF ADMINISTRATION						SIGNATURE
				0800 hrs	1200 hrs	1400 hrs	1800 hrs	2200 hrs	Other Times	
Date	ACICLOVIR	800 mg	ORAL	✓	✓		✓	✓		A. Prescriber

Label

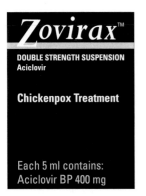

Zovirax™

DOUBLE STRENGTH SUSPENSION
Aciclovir

Chickenpox Treatment

Each 5 ml contains:
Aciclovir BP 400 mg

Exercise 4.44

Prescription

Regular medicines – non-injectable

Date	MEDICINE (Block Letters)	DOSE	ROUTE OF ADMIN	TIMES OF ADMINISTRATION								SIGNATURE
				0800 hrs	1200 hrs	1400 hrs	1800 hrs	2200 hrs	Other Times			
Date	ERYTHROMYCIN	62.5 mg	ORAL	✓	✓		✓	✓				A. Prescriber

Label

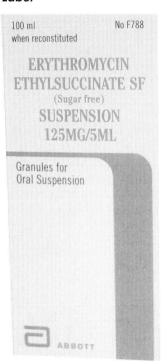

100 ml
when reconstituted

No F788

**ERYTHROMYCIN
ETHYLSUCCINATE SF**
(Sugar free)
**SUSPENSION
125MG/5ML**

Granules for
Oral Suspension

ABBOTT

LEVEL III

Exercise 4.45

Prescription

Regular medicines – non-injectable

| Date | MEDICINE (Block Letters) | DOSE | ROUTE OF ADMIN | TIMES OF ADMINISTRATION | | | | | | | | | SIGNATURE |
				0800 hrs	1200 hrs	1400 hrs	1800 hrs	2200 hrs	Other Times			
Date	ATROPINE	1.2 mg	ORAL					✓				A. Prescriber

Label

> **Atropine Sulphate**
> Tablets BP
> 600 micrograms
>
>
> **28 tablets**

Exercise 4.46

Prescription

Regular medicines – non-injectable

| Date | MEDICINE (Block Letters) | DOSE | ROUTE OF ADMIN | TIMES OF ADMINISTRATION | | | | | | | | | SIGNATURE |
				0800 hrs	1200 hrs	1400 hrs	1800 hrs	2200 hrs	Other Times			
Date	DEXAMETHASONE	500 micrograms	ORAL	✓			✓					A. Prescriber

Label

> **150mL**
>
> **Dexamethasone Solution 2mg/5mL**

Exercise 4.47

Prescription

Regular medicines – non-injectable

Date	MEDICINE (Block Letters)	DOSE	ROUTE OF ADMIN	TIMES OF ADMINISTRATION						SIGNATURE
				0800 hrs	1200 hrs	1400 hrs	1800 hrs	2200 hrs	Other Times	
Date	DORNASE ALFA	2500 units	NEBU-LISER		✓					A. Prescriber

Label

Pulmozyme®

Recombinant human
deoxyribonuclease I
(Dornase alfa)

2,500 Units (2.5 mg)
2.5 ml 1,000 U/ml

30 unit-dose ampoules

⟨Roche⟩

Commentary

- Do not be put off by large numbers
- Take one step at a time making sure you account for all the zeros

Exercise 4.48

Prescription

Regular medicines – non-injectable

Date	MEDICINE (Block Letters)	DOSE	ROUTE OF ADMIN	TIMES OF ADMINISTRATION						SIGNATURE
				0800 hrs	1200 hrs	1400 hrs	1800 hrs	2200 hrs	Other Times	
Date	COLISTIN	1.5 million units	ORAL			✓		✓	0600	A. Prescriber

Label

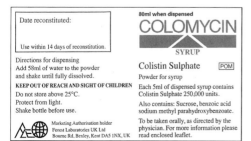

Date reconstituted:

Use within 14 days of reconstitution.

Directions for dispensing
Add 58ml of water to the powder
and shake until fully dissolved.
KEEP OUT OF REACH AND SIGHT OF CHILDREN
Do not store above 25°C.
Protect from light.
Shake bottle before use.

Marketing Authorisation holder
Forest Laboratories UK Ltd
Bourne Rd, Bexley, Kent DA5 1NX, UK

80ml when dispensed
COLOMYCIN
SYRUP

Colistin Sulphate [POM]
Powder for syrup
Each 5ml of dispensed syrup contains
Colistin Sulphate 250,000 units.
Also contains: Sucrose, benzoic acid
sodium methyl parahydroxybenzoate.
To be taken orally, as directed by the
physician. For more information please
read enclosed leaflet.

Exercise 4.49

Prescription

Regular medicines – non-injectable

Date	MEDICINE (Block Letters)	DOSE	ROUTE OF ADMIN	TIMES OF ADMINISTRATION						SIGNATURE
				0800 hrs	1200 hrs	1400 hrs	1800 hrs	2200 hrs	Other Times	
Date	DOMPERIDONE	700 micrograms	ORAL	✓					1600	A. Prescriber

Label

```
200mL



Domperidone
Sugar-free suspension
5mg/5mL
```

Exercise 4.50

Prescription

Regular medicines – non-injectable

Date	MEDICINE (Block Letters)	DOSE	ROUTE OF ADMIN	TIMES OF ADMINISTRATION						SIGNATURE
				0800 hrs	1200 hrs	1400 hrs	1800 hrs	2200 hrs	Other Times	
Date	IODINE	26 mg	ORAL	✓		✓		✓		A. Prescriber

Label

```
100mL

Aqueous Iodine
Oral solution


Total iodine 130mg/mL
```

Exercise 4.51

Prescription

Regular medicines – non-injectable

Date	MEDICINE (Block Letters)	DOSE	ROUTE OF ADMIN	TIMES OF ADMINISTRATION							SIGNATURE
				0800 hrs	1200 hrs	1400 hrs	1800 hrs	2200 hrs	Other Times		
Date	DIGOXIN	75 micrograms	ORAL	✓			✓				A. Prescriber

Label

Lanoxin-PG™ Elixir
Digoxin
**Paediatric/Geriatric
Elixir
50 micrograms
(0.05mg)/ml**

POM

60ml ℮

Exercise 4.52

Prescription

Regular medicines – non-injectable

Date	MEDICINE (Block Letters)	DOSE	ROUTE OF ADMIN	TIMES OF ADMINISTRATION						SIGNATURE
				0800 hrs	1200 hrs	1400 hrs	1800 hrs	2200 hrs	Other Times	
Date	MIRTAZAPINE	22.5 mg	ORAL					✓		A. Prescriber

Label

1 bottle containing 66 ml
**ZISPIN® 15 MG/ML
ORAL SOLUTION**
Mirtazapine
For oral use
1 ml of oral solution contains:
mirtazapine 15 mg

Organon

Exercise 4.53

Prescription

Regular medicines – non-injectable

Date	MEDICINE (Block Letters)	DOSE	ROUTE OF ADMIN	TIMES OF ADMINISTRATION							SIGNATURE
				0800 hrs	1200 hrs	1400 hrs	1800 hrs	2200 hrs	Other Times		
Date	VANCOMYCIN	125 mg	ORAL		✓		✓		0600	2400	A. Prescriber

Label

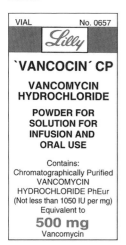

Commentary

● Reconstitute powder by adding 3.8 mL diluent to the vial to make a total volume of 4 mL taking account of the displacement value of 500 mg of vancomycin

Exercise 4.54

Prescription

Regular medicines – non-injectable

Date	MEDICINE (Block Letters)	DOSE	ROUTE OF ADMIN	TIMES OF ADMINISTRATION						SIGNATURE
				0800 hrs	1200 hrs	1400 hrs	1800 hrs	2200 hrs	Other Times	
Date	OSELTAMIVIR	75 mg	ORAL	✓					2000	A. Prescriber

Label

Tamiflu® 12 mg/ml
powder for oral
suspension

Oseltamivir

1 bottle

<Roche>

Exercise 4.55

Prescription

Regular medicines – non-injectable

Date	MEDICINE (Block Letters)	DOSE	ROUTE OF ADMIN	TIMES OF ADMINISTRATION						SIGNATURE
				0800 hrs	1200 hrs	1400 hrs	1800 hrs	2200 hrs	Other Times	
Date	GALANTAMINE	10 mg	ORAL	✓			✓			A. Prescriber

Label

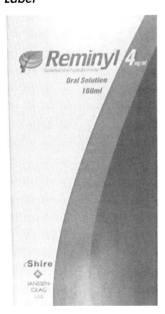

Reminyl 4 mg
Galantamine hydrobromide
Oral Solution
100ml

Shire
◇
JANSSEN-
CILAG
Ltd.

Exercise 4.56

Prescription

Regular medicines – non-injectable

Date	MEDICINE (Block Letters)	DOSE	ROUTE OF ADMIN	TIMES OF ADMINISTRATION						SIGNATURE
				0800 hrs	1200 hrs	1400 hrs	1800 hrs	2200 hrs	Other Times	
Date	PRAMIPEXOLE	264 micrograms	ORAL	Daily in 3 divided doses						A. Prescriber

Label

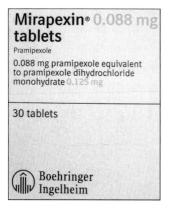

Mirapexin® 0.088 mg
tablets
Pramipexole
0.088 mg pramipexole equivalent
to pramipexole dihydrochloride
monohydrate 0.125 mg

30 tablets

Boehringer
Ingelheim

Some additional calculations to practise now follow in tabular form.

Prescription	Label
4.57 Diflunisal 1 g oral	250 mg tablet
4.58 Lansoprazole 60 mg oral	15 mg capsule
4.59 Hydrocortisone 20 mg oral	10 mg tablet
4.60 Megestrol 80 mg oral	160 mg tablet
4.61 Trimethoprim 200 mg oral	50 mg/5 mL suspension
4.62 Venlafaxine 75 mg oral	37.5 mg tablet
4.63 Amphotericin 150 mg oral	100 mg/1 mL suspension
4.64 Carbamazepine 300 mg oral	100 mg/5 mL suspension
4.65 Cefradine 1 g oral	250 mg/5 mL suspension
4.66 Pizotifen 200 micrograms oral	250 micrograms/5 mL elixir

Dilution of non-parenteral products

Dilution of such products as hydrogen peroxide for use as a mouthwash will not require any calculation.

Two examples of a dilution involving a calculation follow.

EXAMPLE 1

The BNF gives specific guidance on the dilution of potassium permanganate solution. The standard solution is 1 in 1000 (0.1% w/v). A 1 in 10 000 solution is the required strength.

Applying the formula,

$$\frac{Want}{Got} = \frac{1 \text{ in } 10000}{1 \text{ in } 1000}$$

$$= 1 \text{ in } 10$$

The standard solution must be diluted 1 in 10, i.e. 10 mL in 100 mL.

As an alternative, a tablet containing 400 mg (0.4 g) can be dissolved in 4 litres to produce a 0.01% w/v solution.

$$\text{Percentage } w/v = \frac{0.4 \text{ g}}{4000 \text{ mL}} \times 100$$

$$= \frac{0.4 \text{ g}}{4000} \times 100$$

$$= \frac{0.4}{40}$$

$$= \frac{0.4}{40.0} = \frac{4}{400} = \frac{1}{100}$$

or 0.01% w/v

It should not be necessary to dilute antiseptic solutions for topical use. Individual sterile packs are the norm. However, the calculations involved are quite straightforward. It should be noted that this is a calculation involving percentages and so it is necessary to convert milligrams to grams.

EXAMPLE 2

Chlorhexidine is available as a 5% w/v concentrate. In order to produce 1 litre of a 0.05% w/v solution, the calculation is carried out using the formula,

$$\frac{Want \, (\%)}{Got \, (\%)} \times Volume \, (mL) = \begin{array}{l} \text{Volume of concentrated solution required} \\ \text{to be diluted to 1 litre (1000 mL)} \end{array}$$

$$\frac{0.05}{5} \times 1000 = 10 \text{ mL}$$

10 mL of the concentrate must be diluted to 1 litre to produce a 0.05% solution.

CHAPTER 5

Calculating parenteral doses

Small volume injections (up to 20 mL)

Learning outcomes

- Be able to interpret a range of prescriptions of small volume injections
- Be able to interpret a range of labels used for small volume injections
- Understand what is meant by displacement value
- Gain practice/confidence in calculating the quantity to give the patient, using: a) reproduction prescriptions and labels b) the given information in abbreviated form (without prescriptions and labels)

Equipment for measuring the dose

Medicines for injection are presented in either a glass or plastic ampoule (Fig. 5.1) or a rubber-capped vial (Fig. 5.2). The contents are either in the form of a liquid or presented as a powder requiring reconstitution. To aspirate the contents, a syringe and needle of suitable size are selected. Care must be taken to draw up the correct amount into the syringe. It is therefore essential to appreciate the significance of the calibrations on different syringes (Fig. 5.3). The syringe should be held at eye level and there should no longer be any air in the syringe. The reading should be taken at the top of the black bung attached to the plunger of the syringe. When drawing up and giving insulin a syringe (with integral needle) specifically for insulin, calibrated in units must be used (Fig. 5.4).

Overage

When preparing to draw up a parenteral preparation, it should be noted that ampoules containing a solution for injection always contain *more* than the nominal volume. For example, a 1 mL ampoule will normally contain a total volume of 1.1 mL. An overage of 0.1 mL is present so as to allow removal of a full 1 mL dose, otherwise it would not be possible to remove 1 mL due to the 'losses' of injection solution on the internal surfaces of the ampoule. Larger volume ampoules contain overages in proportion to the nominal volume.

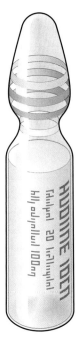

Figure 5.1 Ampoule.

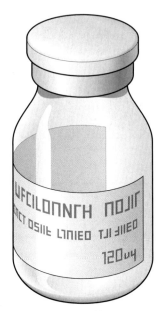

Figure 5.2 Rubber-capped vial.

It follows therefore that it is very important to measure all doses and not simply to draw up the contents of the ampoule. The presence of overages in ampoules is one reason why it is not acceptable to measure doses in terms of, for example, half an ampoule. A nominal 1 mL ampoule that contains 10 mg per 1 mL will contain 11 mg in 1.1 mL. Giving a dose of half the contents of the ampoule or the full content of the ampoule could introduce a drug error. In practical terms, nurses need to be aware of overages but rarely will significant problems be created by the presence of an overage. There is no substitute for measuring the dose accurately. It should be noted that labels of Controlled Drugs show the presence of an overage for legal reasons.

Displacement values

A number of drugs are unstable in solution and are therefore supplied in powder form. Prior to administration, the powder must be reconstituted using a diluent (or solvent). Water for Injections is commonly used but sodium chloride 0.9% solution may be the recommended diluent; on occasion, a specially formulated diluent may be provided. The product data sheet should be consulted for detailed information. Enough liquid is needed to dissolve the contents to produce a concentration that prevents irritation of body tissues but at the same time is of minimum volume so as to make the injection less painful.

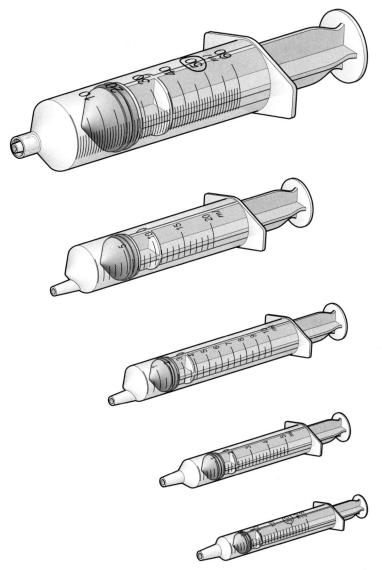

Figure 5.3 Syringes showing different calibrations.

The addition of 5 mL of a diluent to a vial containing 500 mg of a drug in powder form will produce a volume of *more* than 5 mL due to the effect of the powder (Fig. 5.5). It will be seen in Fig. 5.5 that the powder has added 0.2 mL to the volume of diluent added. This is the displacement value (DV). If the dose to be administered is *less* than 500 mg, it will be important to take account of the displacement value.

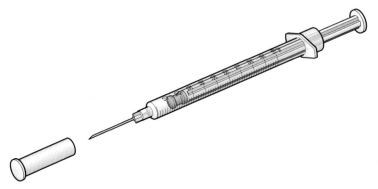

Figure 5.4 Insulin syringe showing calibrations.

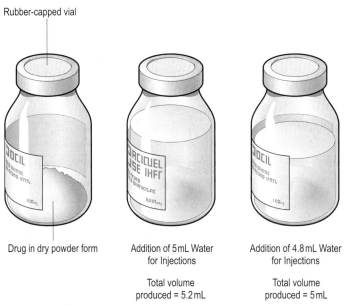

Rubber-capped vial

Drug in dry powder form | Addition of 5 mL Water for Injections | Addition of 4.8 mL Water for Injections

Total volume produced = 5.2 mL | Total volume produced = 5 mL

Figure 5.5 Displacement of liquid when reconstituting an injection.

Staying with this example, a dose of 250 mg of a drug is to be administered from the 500 mg vial. The contents of the vial of 500 mg displace 0.2 mL of diluent. It is therefore necessary to add to the vial 5 mL minus 0.2 mL, which equals 4.8 mL, to produce a total volume of solution of 5 mL. The resulting solution contains 500 mg in 5 mL.

To obtain the required dose, the usual formula can then be applied:

$\dfrac{\text{Want}}{\text{Got}} \times \text{Volume (mL)} = \text{Volume in mL to be given}$

$$= \dfrac{250}{500} \times 5$$
$$= 2.5\,\text{mL}$$

If allowance is *not* made for the DV, measuring and administering a dose of 2.5 mL would result in a drug error.

Thus, if 5 mL of a diluent was added (not taking account of the DV), a total volume of 5.2 mL would be produced. The dose of 250 mg would be contained in:

$$\dfrac{250}{500} \times 5.2\,\text{mL} = 2.6\,\text{mL}$$

Displacement values will normally be found in the product literature. If for some reason the DV is not known, a suitable volume of diluent is added to the vial in the usual way and the powder fully dissolved. The total contents of the vial are measured by drawing into a syringe. The required dose can then be calculated.

It is important to note that all powders intended to be reconstituted before use will displace a certain volume of diluent. Powder for colomycin syrup displaces 22 mL of water when made up to the required volume of 80 mL, i.e. 58 mL of water must be added to produce a final volume of 80 mL.

How to calculate the quantity to give of small volume injections

Interpretation of the prescription and the label of a parenteral preparation requires the same principles to be followed as for a non-parenteral preparation.

The following pages (pp. 102–109) contain fully worked-up examples which demonstrate how to calculate doses of small volume parenteral drugs. Included are examples of calculations at the levels of complexity described in Chapter 3. (Practice exercises are provided on pp. 110–121. Answers to these are given on p. 149.)

A standard format is used which includes the given information, namely the prescription and the label; a commentary intended to provide additional information; the workings involved; and finally, what the patient will be given on each occasion.

For various technical reasons, it has not been possible to reproduce some labels. In such cases, facsimile labels have been created. Although it is recognised that dispensing from bulk packs is avoided where possible, there may still be occasions where this is done.

The examples shown are based on current practice. It is important, however, to note that, as it is beyond the scope of this book to give details of the patients' clinical condition, the doses should be regarded as illustrative only.

No calculation required

Example 5.1

Prescription

Regular medicines – injectable

Date	MEDICINE (Block Letters)	DOSE	ROUTE OF ADMIN	TIMES OF ADMINISTRATION						SIGNATURE
				0800 hrs	1200 hrs	1400 hrs	1800 hrs	2200 hrs	Other Times	
Date	RANITIDINE	50 mg	IM	✓		✓		✓		A. Prescriber

Label

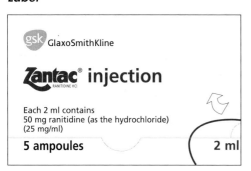

Commentary

● No calculation is involved here since the prescribed dose corresponds to the strength on the label

The patient will be given:
2 mL IM injection

LEVEL I

Example 5.2

Prescription

Once only medicines – all routes

Date	MEDICINE	DOSE	ROUTE OF ADMIN	TIME OF ADMIN	SIGNATURE
Date	PROTIRELIN	200 micrograms	IV	1100 hrs	A. Prescriber

Label

> **Protirelin Injection**
> **100 micrograms/mL**
>
> 2mL ampoule

Commentary

● A straightforward example
● No need for formula

Workings

The prescribed dose is *more* than the amount contained in 1 mL.

If there are 100 micrograms in 1 mL, then 200 micrograms equals 2 mL.

The patient will be given:
2 mL IV injection

Example 5.3

Prescription

Regular medicines – injectable

Date	MEDICINE (Block Letters)	DOSE	ROUTE OF ADMIN	0800 hrs	1200 hrs	1400 hrs	1800 hrs	2200 hrs	Other Times		SIGNATURE
					TIMES OF ADMINISTRATION						
Date	DICLOFENAC	75 mg	IM		✓						A. Prescriber

Label

> **Diclofenac Injection 25mg/1mL**
>
> 3mL ampoule

Commentary

- This is another straightforward example
- If in doubt, use the formula

Workings

The prescribed dose is *more* than the amount contained in 1 mL.

Applying the formula,

$$\frac{\text{Want}}{\text{Got}} \times \text{Volume}$$

$$= \frac{75\,\text{mg}}{25\,\text{mg}} \times 1\,\text{mL}$$

$$= \frac{\overset{3}{\cancel{75}}\,\cancel{\text{mg}}}{\underset{1}{\cancel{25}}\,\cancel{\text{mg}}} \times 1\,\text{mL}$$

$$= 3\,\text{mL}$$

The patient will be given:
3 mL IM injection

LEVEL II

Example 5.4

Prescription

Once only medicines – all routes

Date	MEDICINE	DOSE	ROUTE OF ADMIN	TIME OF ADMIN	SIGNATURE
Date	*PHYTOMENADIONE*	*1 mg*	*IM*	*1205 hrs*	*A. Prescriber*

Label

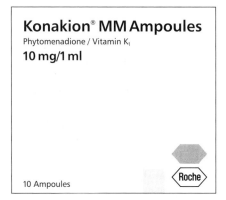

Konakion® MM Ampoules
Phytomenadione / Vitamin K₁
10 mg/1 ml

10 Ampoules   ⟨Roche⟩

Commentary

● Take time when working with decimals
● If in doubt, use the formula
● Stick to the rules of arithmetic

Workings
The prescribed dose is *less* than the amount contained in 1 mL.

Applying the formula,

$$\frac{\text{Want}}{\text{Got}} \times \text{Volume}$$

$$= \frac{1\,\text{mg}}{10\,\text{mg}} \times 1\,\text{mL}$$

$$= \frac{1\,\cancel{\text{mg}}}{10\,\cancel{\text{mg}}} \times 1\,\text{mL}$$

$$= \frac{1}{10}\,\text{mL}$$

$$= 10\overline{)\,1.0\,}^{\,0.1}$$

$$= 0.1\,\text{mL}$$

The patient will be given:
0.1 mL IM injection

Example 5.5

Prescription

Once only medicines – all routes

Date	MEDICINE	DOSE	ROUTE OF ADMIN	TIME OF ADMIN	SIGNATURE
Date	PAPAVERETUM	3.85 mg	IM	0035 hrs	A. Prescriber

Label

> **Papaveretum Injection 15.4mg/mL**
>
> 1mL ampoule
>
> **CD**

Commentary

- This is a Controlled Drug
- It is always safer to work in whole numbers
- Make sure you move the decimal point the same number of places to the right above and below the line
- This is an occasion when you would be advised to use a calculator to divide 385 by 1540
- Note that the ampoules contain a declared overage of 0.1 mL

Workings

The prescribed dose is *less* than the amount contained in 1 mL.

Applying the formula,

$$\frac{\text{Want}}{\text{Got}} \times \text{Volume}$$

$$= \frac{3.85\,\text{mg}}{15.4\,\text{mg}} \times 1\,\text{mL}$$

$$= \frac{3.85\,\text{mg}}{15.40\,\text{mg}} \times 1\,\text{mL}$$

$$= \frac{385}{1540}\,\text{mL}$$

$$= \frac{77}{308}\,\text{mL}$$

$$= \frac{1}{4}\,\text{mL}$$

$$= 0.25\,\text{mL}$$

The patient will be given:

0.25 mL IM injection

Example 5.6

Prescription

Regular medicines – injectable

Date	MEDICINE (Block Letters)	DOSE	ROUTE OF ADMIN	TIMES OF ADMINISTRATION							SIGNATURE
				0800 hrs	1200 hrs	1400 hrs	1800 hrs	2200 hrs	Other Times	
Date	BENZATROPINE	750 micrograms	IM	✓	Repeated if symptoms reappear after discussion with prescriber					A. Prescriber

Label

Benzatropine
Injection
1mg/mL

10 × 2mL ampoules

Commentary

● The prescription and the label are in different units and so first a conversion is needed

Workings
The dose available is 1 mg/1 mL, which is the same as 1000 micrograms/1 mL.

Applying the formula,

$$\frac{\text{Want}}{\text{Got}} \times \text{Volume}$$

$$= \frac{750 \text{ micrograms}}{1000 \text{ micrograms}} \times 1 \text{mL}$$

$$= \frac{75\cancel{0} \text{ micrograms}}{100\cancel{0} \text{ micrograms}} \times 1 \text{mL}$$

$$= \frac{75}{100} \text{mL}$$

$$= 0.75 \text{mL}$$

The patient will be given:
0.75 mL IM injection

Example 5.7

Prescription

Once only medicines – all routes

Date	MEDICINE	DOSE	ROUTE OF ADMIN	TIME OF ADMIN	SIGNATURE
Date	DESMOPRESSIN	400 nanograms	SC	0855 hrs	A. Prescriber

Label

1 ml
DDAVP/
DESMOPRESSIN
Injection iv., i.m. or s.c.
Desmopressin acetate
4 mcg in 1 ml
FERRING
PHARMACEUTICALS

Commentary

● The prescription and the label are in different units
● Working with nanograms calls for the utmost care

Workings

First, convert 4 micrograms to nanograms:

4×1000 [1000 nanograms

in 1 microgram]

$= 4000$ nanograms

Applying the formula,

$$\frac{Want}{Got} \times Volume$$

$$= \frac{400 \text{ nanograms}}{4000 \text{ nanograms}} \times 1 \text{mL}$$

$$= \frac{4\cancel{00} \text{ nanograms}}{4\cancel{000} \text{ nanograms}} \times 1 \text{mL}$$

$$= \frac{4}{40} \text{ mL}$$

$$= \frac{1}{10} \text{ mL}$$

$$= 0.1 \text{ml}$$

The patient will be given:

0.1 mL SC injection

LEVEL III

Example 5.8

Prescription

Once only medicines – all routes

Date	MEDICINE	DOSE	ROUTE OF ADMIN	TIME OF ADMIN	SIGNATURE
Date	LORAZEPAM	25 micrograms/kg	IM	2000 hrs	A. Prescriber

Label

Lorazepam Injection 4mg/mL

1mL ampoule

Commentary

● The patient weighs 70 kg
● In most cases, the prescriber will already have worked out the dose to be given
● Nurses should, however, know how this is done and be prepared to challenge the prescriber if in doubt

Workings

For a 70 kg patient, the dose required is

70 × 25 micrograms
= 1750 micrograms

The strength available is 4 mg/mL, which is the same as 4000 micrograms/mL.

The prescribed dose is *less* than the amount contained in 1 mL.

Applying the formula,

$$\frac{\text{Want}}{\text{Got}} \times \text{Volume}$$

$$= \frac{1750 \text{ micrograms}}{4000 \text{ micrograms}} \times 1\text{mL}$$

$$= \frac{175\cancel{0} \text{ micrograms}}{400\cancel{0} \text{ micrograms}} \times 1\text{mL}$$

$$= \frac{175}{400} \text{ mL}$$

$$= \frac{7}{16}$$

$$= 16\overline{)7.000}^{\,0.437}$$

$$= 0.437$$

$$\approx 0.44 \text{ mL}$$

The patient will be given:
0.44 mL IM injection

Example 5.9

Prescription

Once only medicines – all routes

Date	MEDICINE	DOSE	ROUTE OF ADMIN	TIME OF ADMIN	SIGNATURE
Date	INDOMETACIN	200 micrograms/kg	IV	0800 hrs	A. Prescriber
Date	INDOMETACIN	250 micrograms/kg	IV	2000 hrs	A. Prescriber

Label

Indometacin
(Indomethacin)

PDA
For IV injection
1 mg vial powder for reconstitution

3 x 1 mg vials

Commentary

● The patient weighs 3.5 kg
● The product literature states that 2 mL of Water for Injections should be used to dilute
● The label gives the abbreviation PDA indicating the therapeutic use of this drug
● Note the change in spelling of the approved name

Workings

First dose

Multiply prescribed dose by patient's weight,

200 micrograms × 3.5
= 700 micrograms

Applying the formula,

$$\frac{Want}{Got} \times Volume$$

$$= \frac{700 \text{ micrograms}}{1000 \text{ micrograms (i.e. 1 mg)}} \times 2 \text{ mL}$$

$$= \frac{14}{10} \text{ mL}$$

$$= 1.4 \text{ mL}$$

The patient will be given:
First dose: 1.4 mL IV injection

Second dose

Multiply prescribed dose by patient's weight,

250 micrograms × 3.5
= 875 micrograms

Applying the formula,

$$\frac{Want}{Got} \times Volume$$

$$= \frac{875 \text{ micrograms}}{1000 \text{ micrograms}} \times 2 \text{ mL}$$

$$= \frac{875}{500} \text{ mL}$$

$$= 1.75 \text{ mL}$$

Second dose: 1.75 mL IV injection

Practice exercises (answers on pp. 149–150)

LEVEL I

Exercise 5.1

Prescription

Once only medicines – all routes

Date	MEDICINE	DOSE	ROUTE OF ADMIN	TIME OF ADMIN	SIGNATURE
Date	BETAMETHASONE SODIUM PHOSPHATE	1 mg	IM	1440 hrs	A. Prescriber

Label

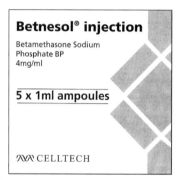

Exercise 5.2

Prescription

Once only medicines – all routes

Date	MEDICINE	DOSE	ROUTE OF ADMIN	TIME OF ADMIN	SIGNATURE
Date	NALOXONE HYDROCHLORIDE	100 micrograms	IV	0545 hrs	A. Prescriber

Label

Naloxone hydrochloride Injection 400 micrograms/mL

Exercise 5.3

Prescription

Once only medicines – all routes

Date	MEDICINE	DOSE	ROUTE OF ADMIN	TIME OF ADMIN	SIGNATURE
Date	FUROSEMIDE	10 mg	IM	1045 hrs	A. Prescriber

Label

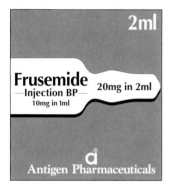

Exercise 5.4

Prescription

Once only medicines – all routes

Date	MEDICINE	DOSE	ROUTE OF ADMIN	TIME OF ADMIN	SIGNATURE
Date	FUROSEMIDE	2 mg	IV	2150 hrs	A. Prescriber

Label

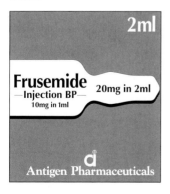

LEVEL II

Exercise 5.5

Prescription

Once only medicines – all routes

Date	MEDICINE	DOSE	ROUTE OF ADMIN	TIME OF ADMIN	SIGNATURE
Date	GLYCOPYRRONIUM BROMIDE	300 micrograms	IM	0900 hrs	A. Prescriber

Label

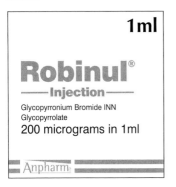

1ml

Robinul®
——Injection——

Glycopyrronium Bromide INN
Glycopyrrolate
200 micrograms in 1ml

Anpharm

Exercise 5.6

Prescription

Once only medicines – all routes

Date	MEDICINE	DOSE	ROUTE OF ADMIN	TIME OF ADMIN	SIGNATURE
Date	ATROPINE SULPHATE	400 micrograms	IM	0800 hrs	A. Prescriber

Label

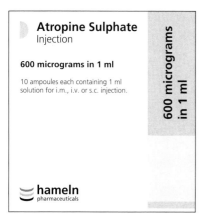

Atropine Sulphate
Injection

600 micrograms in 1 ml

10 ampoules each containing 1 ml
solution for i.m., i.v. or s.c. injection.

600 micrograms in 1 ml

hameln
pharmaceuticals

Exercise 5.7

Prescription

Regular medicines – injectable

Date	MEDICINE (Block Letters)	DOSE	ROUTE OF ADMIN	TIMES OF ADMINISTRATION						SIGNATURE
				0800 hrs	1200 hrs	1400 hrs	1800 hrs	2200 hrs	Other Times	
Date	BUPRENORPHINE	450 micrograms	IV	✓		✓		✓		A. Prescriber

Label

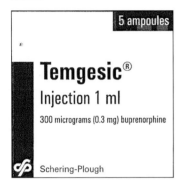

Exercise 5.8

Prescription

Once only medicines – all routes

Date	MEDICINE	DOSE	ROUTE OF ADMIN	TIME OF ADMIN	SIGNATURE
Date	DIAZEPAM EMULSION	7.5 mg	IV	30 min. prior to procedure	A. Prescriber

Label

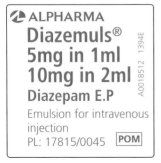

Exercise 5.9

Prescription

Regular medicines – injectable

Date	MEDICINE (Block Letters)	DOSE	ROUTE OF ADMIN	TIMES OF ADMINISTRATION							SIGNATURE
				0800 hrs	1200 hrs	1400 hrs	1800 hrs	2200 hrs	Other Times	
Date	NEOSTIGMINE	1 mg	SC	✓	✓	✓	✓	✓		A. Prescriber

Label

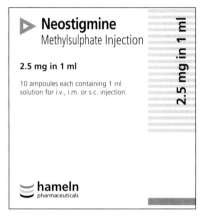

Neostigmine
Methylsulphate Injection

2.5 mg in 1 ml

10 ampoules each containing 1 ml
solution for i.v., i.m. or s.c. injection.

2.5 mg in 1 ml

hameln
pharmaceuticals

Exercise 5.10

Prescription

Once only medicines – all routes

Date	MEDICINE	DOSE	ROUTE OF ADMIN	TIME OF ADMIN	SIGNATURE
Date	SALBUTAMOL	125 micrograms	Slow IV	1320 hrs	A. Prescriber

Label

**Salbutamol
Injection
500 micrograms/mL**

1mL ampoule

Exercise 5.11

Prescription

Regular medicines – injectable

Date	MEDICINE (Block Letters)	DOSE	ROUTE OF ADMIN	TIMES OF ADMINISTRATION						SIGNATURE
				0800 hrs	1200 hrs	1400 hrs	1800 hrs	2200 hrs	Other Times	
Date	CALCITRIOL	1.5 micrograms	IV		✓	Mondays Wednesdays Fridays				A. Prescriber

Label

Calcitriol
Injection
2 micrograms/mL

1mL amp.

Exercise 5.12

Prescription

Regular medicines – injectable

Date	MEDICINE (Block Letters)	DOSE	ROUTE OF ADMIN	TIMES OF ADMINISTRATION						SIGNATURE
				0800 hrs	1200 hrs	1400 hrs	1800 hrs	2200 hrs	Other Times	
Date	CEFOTAXIME	150 mg	IV	✓	✓		✓	✓		A. Prescriber

Label

Cefotaxime
Injection
500mg/2mL vial
powder for reconstitution

500mg vial

Commentary

● Note, 2 mL is the final volume taking into account the displacement value

Exercise 5.13

Prescription

Once only medicines – all routes

Date	MEDICINE	DOSE	ROUTE OF ADMIN	TIME OF ADMIN	SIGNATURE
Date	EDROPHONIUM CHLORIDE	2 mg	IV	1430 hrs	A. Prescriber
	then if no adverse reaction after 30 seconds				
Date	EDROPHONIUM CHLORIDE	8 mg	IV		A. Prescriber

Label

**Edrophonium chloride
Injection
10mg/mL**

1mL ampoule

LEVEL III

Exercise 5.14

Prescription

Regular medicines – injectable

Date	MEDICINE (Block Letters)	DOSE	ROUTE OF ADMIN	TIMES OF ADMINISTRATION						SIGNATURE
				0800 hrs	1200 hrs	1400 hrs	1800 hrs	2200 hrs	Other Times	
Date	HEPARIN	5000 units	SC	✓			✓			A. Prescriber

Label

**Heparin (Mucous)
Injection B.P.
25,000 Units/ml**
heparin sodium

5 vials of 5 ml

PL 0043/0039R
PA 46/36/3 **POM**

Exercise 5.15

Prescription

Once only medicines – all routes

Date	MEDICINE	DOSE	ROUTE OF ADMIN	TIME OF ADMIN	SIGNATURE
Date	ADRENALINE	250 micrograms	IM	1710 hrs	A. Prescriber

Label

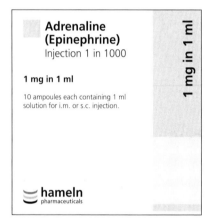

Adrenaline (Epinephrine)
Injection 1 in 1000

1 mg in 1 ml

10 ampoules each containing 1 ml solution for i.m. or s.c. injection.

1 mg in 1 ml

hameln pharmaceuticals

Commentary

● Adrenaline injection is supplied as strength 1 in 1000, which means 1 mg in 1 mL
● 1 mg is the same as 1000 micrograms

Exercise 5.16

Prescription

Regular medicines – injectable

Date	MEDICINE (Block Letters)	DOSE	ROUTE OF ADMIN	TIMES OF ADMINISTRATION						SIGNATURE
				0800 hrs	1200 hrs	1400 hrs	1800 hrs	2200 hrs	Other Times	
Date	PETHIDINE	1 mg/kg	IM	Every 4 hours						A. Prescriber

Label

Pethidine Injection 50mg in 1mL

10 ampoules

Commentary

● This is a Controlled Drug
● The patient's weight is 20 kg
● For every kg of body weight, 1 mg is to be given
● These ampoules would normally contain a declared overage of 0.1 mL

Exercise 5.17

Prescription

Regular medicines – injectable

Date	MEDICINE (Block Letters)	DOSE	ROUTE OF ADMIN	TIMES OF ADMINISTRATION						SIGNATURE
				0800 hrs	1200 hrs	1400 hrs	1800 hrs	2200 hrs	Other Times	
Date	GANCICLOVIR	5 mg/kg	IV	✓						A. Prescriber

Label

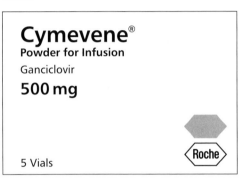

Cymevene®
Powder for Infusion
Ganciclovir
500 mg

5 Vials ⟨Roche⟩

Commentary

● The patient weighs 60 kg
● The IV powder has to be reconstituted. Assume that 10 mL is the volume after Water for Injections has been added

Exercise 5.18

Prescription

Once only medicines – all routes

Date	MEDICINE	DOSE	ROUTE OF ADMIN	TIME OF ADMIN	SIGNATURE
Date	ADRENALINE (epinephrine)	500 micrograms	IM	1840 hrs	A. Prescriber

Label

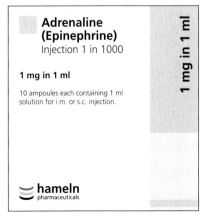

Adrenaline (Epinephrine)
Injection 1 in 1000

1 mg in 1 ml

10 ampoules each containing 1 ml
solution for i.m. or s.c. injection.

1 mg in 1 ml

hameln
pharmaceuticals

Exercise 5.19

Prescription

Once only medicines – all routes

Date	MEDICINE	DOSE	ROUTE OF ADMIN	TIME OF ADMIN	SIGNATURE
Date	MAGNESIUM SULPHATE	2 g	IV	0750 hrs	A. Prescriber
		Dilute to 10% w/v strength before using			

Label

```
2ml
Magnesium
Sulphate
Injection
50% w/v 1g in 2ml

For IM or IV use
CELLTECH
POM

PL 00039/5903R        81490
```

Commentary

- Calculate amount of injection and the dilution required

Exercise 5.20

Prescription

Once only medicines – all routes

Date	MEDICINE	DOSE	ROUTE OF ADMIN	TIME OF ADMIN	SIGNATURE
Date	HYOSCINE	2.4 mg	IM	0830 hrs	A. Prescriber

Label

```
Hyoscine hydrobromide
Injection
600 micrograms/mL

5 ampoules
```

Exercise 5.21

Prescription

Once only medicines – all routes

Date	MEDICINE	DOSE	ROUTE OF ADMIN	TIME OF ADMIN	SIGNATURE
Date	PHENYLEPHRINE	200 micrograms	IV	1210 hrs	A. Prescriber

Label

```
Phenylephrine 1%
Injection
10mg/mL


1mL ampoule
```

Some additional calculations to practise now follow in tabular form.

Prescription	Label
5.22 Methadone 7.5 mg SC	10 mg/mL injection
5.23 Sodium aurothiomalate 10 mg IM	20 mg/mL injection
5.24 Triamcinolone 2.5 mg intra-articular injection	10 mg/mL injection
5.25 Salbutamol 125 micrograms slow IV	250 micrograms/mL injection
5.26 Ondansetron 8 mg IM	2 mg/mL injection

Syringe driver

The syringe driver is designed to provide a steady infusion of drugs over a 24 hour period. It may be used to administer medication by the subcutaneous (SC), intravenous (IV), epidural, intra-arterial, intramuscular, intrathecal and nasogastric routes. Most commonly used are the SC and IV routes; a burette and pump may be preferred for other routes. Most syringe drivers are small, lightweight, battery-operated and portable. The syringe rests on a syringe barrel holder and is fixed in place.

Being simply another type of delivery system, the syringe driver presents no more difficulty than calculations by any other route. As much care is required in reading the prescription and the details on the label as when preparing to administer any other medicine. The amount of diluent is dependent on the number and volume of the drugs to be delivered.

Once the syringe is filled with the appropriate amount of drug(s) and diluent, it is attached to an infusion set designed for the purpose. The set is then primed using some of the contents (1 mL in fact) of the syringe. When using the SC route, the infusion set should have a previously attached plastic cannula or 'butterfly' needle; for the IV route, the infusion set, once primed, is attached to an already sited IV cannula. When the syringe is filled, the tubing primed and the needle/cannula in place/attached, the rate the plunger is to advance must be set in accordance with the prescription.

The size of syringe is 5 mL, 10 mL, 20 mL or 30 mL.

Syringe drivers are available that can be set at:

● *either* millimetres per hour (for rapid infusions)
● *or* millimetres per 24 hours (for palliative care)

In the interests of patient safety, standardisation has been encouraged and health authorities have been opting for one or other of these types. It should be noted that these settings express the *distance* travelled by the plunger within a span of time, and not the volume of drug.

If both types of syringe drivers are available, great care must be taken when setting up, since a 24-fold error can occur.

For convenience, the volume of drug(s) and diluent should be made up to 48 mm.

To set the rate:

1. Measure the distance the plunger has to travel from the first line on the syringe to the black rubber bung of the plunger.
2. Dial this amount on the syringe driver.
3. Fill the connecting tubing (the first syringe will run through 1–2 hours early but subsequent syringes will run on time).
4. Insert battery into driver.
5. Press start/test or boost button once.
   (after Reynard, Kindlen & Aport 2004).

It is good practice once the infusion has commenced to check within the first half-hour that the plunger is proceeding as intended and that the patient is comfortable. A check thereafter at least every 4 hours should suffice unless local policy dictates otherwise.

A syringe pump is a separate device in which the rate of flow is controlled by the speed of the piston attached to the syringe plunger. Highly concentrated drugs may be administered intravenously by this method, usually via a 60 mL syringe. The rate is set in millilitres per hour. Syringe pumps are more likely to be used in intensive care situations.

Large volume parenterals (more than 20 mL)

Learning outcomes

- Be able to interpret prescriptions for large volume parenteral products
- Recognise the range and presentation of solutions used for intravenous infusion
- Be able to interpret the information given on infusion solution containers and relevant data sheet
- Know the rates at which intravenous infusions are delivered by different types of administration set
- Be able to calculate the dilution of parenteral drugs prior to administration/use
- Be able to calculate the rate of flow in millilitres per hour (mL/h) for an intravenous infusion
- Know how to key the correct information into an infusion pump
- Gain practice/confidence in calculating flow rates using the given information in abbreviated form (without prescriptions and labels)

Intravenous infusion

The administration of intravenous fluids carries with it considerable risk in terms of the volume of fluid infused, the content of the fluid and the rate at which the fluid is infused. As a result, extreme care is required at the start of an infusion, during the time it is being infused and whenever there is a changeover of fluid or a change in the fluid regime.

The principles of checking apply in exactly the same way as for the administration of any medication.

First, you should read the prescription. It *must* show the:

- date
- name of the infusion fluid (including strength/dose) and any additives
- volume to be infused
- route of administration
- duration of administration
- prescriber's signature

If any one of these is missing, the prescription must be referred back to the prescriber.

Nurses have to be ready to interpret common abbreviations and chemical symbols used by some prescribers. These include:

IV	intravenous
IVI	intravenous infusion
mL	millilitre
h	hour
Na$^+$ Cl$^-$	sodium chloride
K$^+$ Cl$^-$	potassium chloride

It should be noted that where there is more than one intravenous line in use, a separate prescription should be used for each line.

The correct bag of solution must then be selected.

Extreme care is required at all times in comparing the details of the solution on the prescription with the details of the solution on the bag. Many combinations of solution are available. It is essential not only to select the correct solution but also to ensure that it is of the prescribed strength. The strength is expressed as a percentage. All percentage solutions are expressed as weight in volume (w/v). The most commonly used solutions are single preparations, such as:

● Sodium chloride 0.9% (Fig. 5.6) (other strengths are available, e.g. 0.18%)
● Glucose 5% (Fig. 5.7) (other strengths are available, e.g. 10%)

Numerous ready-mixed solutions containing more than one substance are available. Some examples are listed below.

● Sodium chloride 0.18% and glucose 4%
● Potassium chloride 0.3%, sodium chloride 0.18% and glucose 4%
● Potassium chloride 0.2%, sodium chloride 0.18% and glucose 4%
● Potassium chloride 0.2% and sodium chloride 0.9% (Fig. 5.8)
● Potassium chloride 0.3% and glucose 5%
● Potassium chloride 0.15% and glucose 10%
● Sodium chloride 0.9%, potassium chloride 20 mmol/L and magnesium sulphate 8 mmol/L

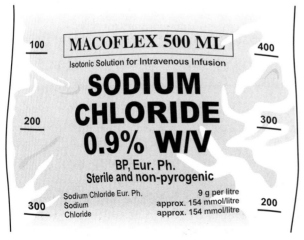

Figure 5.6 Sodium chloride 0.9% infusion label.

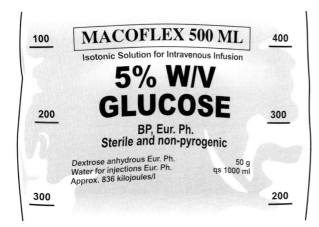

Figure 5.7 Glucose 5% infusion label.

These figures may appear complex but this does not need to cause any difficulty as long as both the prescription and the label *match* in every detail.

Time should be taken by two appropriately qualified members of staff to read out the details together on the prescription and ensure that they correspond precisely with the details on the bag prior to administration. The implications of making an error with intravenous therapy are major. No matter what is being administered, the need to be absolutely certain that the patient is receiving the intended solution in the correct volume at the correct rate is paramount.

The utmost care must be taken when infusing a solution containing potassium chloride. If concentrated potassium chloride solution is inadequately mixed or a depletion of potassium is treated too rapidly, there is a high risk of cardiac arrest. For this reason, wherever possible, a ready-prepared infusion should be used (see Fig. 5.8). In the event of potassium having to be added by clinical staff, special procedures will be in place which must be adhered to.

The information on a typical intravenous infusion bag is shown in Fig. 5.6.

● The volumes in common use are 1000 mL, 500 mL, 250 mL, 100 mL and 50 mL
● The administration time of the prescribed fluid is normally expressed in numbers of hours
● Common frequencies are 6 hourly, 8 hourly, 12 hourly
● Small volumes may be prescribed for administration over a number of minutes, e.g. 10 min, 30 min

Infusions require to be infused via an administration set which relays the fluid from the bag to a cannula already sited in a vein. Administration sets vary depending on whether the infusion is to be administered by gravity or by pump and whether the infusion is of a clear fluid or of blood. It is essential to select the appropriate set as the rate of flow has been predetermined in the different types available.

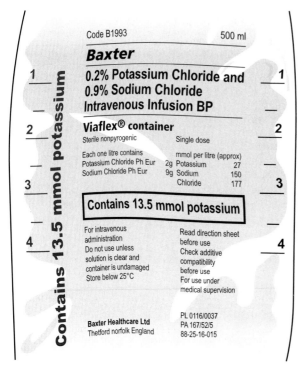

Figure 5.8 Potassium chloride 0.2% and sodium chloride 0.9% infusion label.

For adults, the set to use for:

● all clear solutions, is one that delivers at 20 drops/mL
● blood and blood components, because they are more viscous (thicker), is one that delivers at 15 drops/mL

If there is any doubt about which set to use, reference should be made to the administration set packaging.

The safest way to administer an intravenous infusion is to deliver it via an infusion pump, as this method provides very precise control over the rate of the fluid. Where large volumes are to be given or where the fluid and/or its contents are highly potent, the standard expected would involve the use of an infusion pump. However, infusion pumps are costly, and it may not be possible to provide one in every case. It is obvious therefore that nurses require to be competent in managing infusions with or without an infusion pump.

GRAVITY-ASSISTED INFUSION

An infusion may be set up which simply allows the fluid to travel from the bag through the administration set to the cannula under the influence of gravity. With this type of infusion, the rate of fluid can be controlled in three ways. These are the:

- aperture within the drip chamber (preset in drops per mL)
- roller clamp (controlled manually)
- height of the bag (the higher the infusion stand is set, the faster the rate)

To calculate how to set the infusion at the prescribed rate, you require to know the amount to be infused and the length of time the infusion is to take. The next step is to work out how much will be infused in 1 hour. This is done by dividing the total volume by the time the infusion is to take:

$$\text{Number of mL per hour (mL/h)} = \frac{\text{Total volume}}{\text{Duration}}$$

For example, 500 mL of a clear fluid is to be transfused over 4 hours:

$$\text{mL/h} = \frac{500\,\text{mL}}{4}$$
$$= 125\,\text{mL}$$

The prescribed rate is 125 mL/h.

In order that the infusion can be regulated, however, the nurse needs to know how many drops per minute at which to set the infusion. In this instance, a clear solution is in use and therefore the appropriate administration set would be one set at 20 drops/mL.

To calculate the rate of flow in drops per minute, which the nurse will be able to count using a watch:

$$\text{Drops/min} = \frac{\text{Volume of fluid in mL} \times 20}{\text{Duration in min}}$$
$$= \frac{500 \times 20}{4 \times 60}$$
$$= \frac{500}{12}$$
$$= 41.66 \text{ rep.}$$
$$= 42 \text{ (to nearest whole number)}$$

The infusion can be controlled at 42 drops per minute.

Health authority prescription sheets may provide a ready reckoner to assist the nurse in calculating the rate of flow and should be used where provided.

Since other variables come into play, such as the positioning of the patient, which may increase the flow rate, this method is not wholly reliable, and so to limit the risks associated with the infusion of large volumes of fluid, the maximum size of bag used is 500 mL.

PUMP-ASSISTED INFUSION

When using an infusion pump (Fig. 5.9), the appropriate administration set (specifically for use with a pump) must be used.

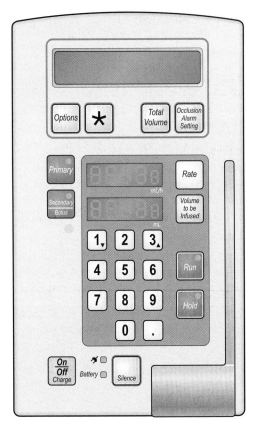

Figure 5.9 Infusion pump.

The infusion pump has been designed to provide very precise control of the rate at which the fluid is infused. It does not serve the purpose of a calculator and so it is essential to know how to calculate what the patient is to receive, i.e. the flow rate. This is expressed in millilitres per hour (mL/h).

Once the calculation has been made, and only then, the rate and the total volume the patient is to receive can be keyed in to the pump.

To calculate the flow rate, the prescribed volume (always in mL) is divided by the duration of the infusion (always per hour):

$$\text{Flow rate} = \frac{\text{Total volume (mL)}}{\text{Duration (h)}}$$

If a *volume* of 1000 mL is to be infused over 8 hours, it can be represented as:

$$\frac{1000\,\text{mL}}{8} = 125\,\text{mL}$$

The *rate* is therefore 125 mL per hour.

These figures are then carefully entered using the appropriate keys. The pump will not correct any errors made; it will only perform on the basis of the information that has been entered into it. Over-reliance on it is to be avoided and periodic checks (e.g. hourly) must be made to ensure that the amount infused and the amount left, when added together, are the same as the original volume to be infused.

Dilution of parenteral medicines

In current clinical practice, in addition to calculating flow rates, it may be necessary to calculate how to dilute a solution to give a lower concentration of a drug in the solution suitable for intravenous infusion. Preparations should normally be provided in a ready-to-use form from the pharmacy so as to reduce the risk of error and microbial contamination.

Dilution prior to use may be necessary, however, in some clinical settings, especially when administering irritant solutions intravenously. The BNF lists injections that require dilution prior to use. The diluents to be used (in order to avoid chemical incompatibility) are always specified. Examples of parenteral products that require dilution before administration are as follows:

● aclarubicin
● amphotericin
● carboplatin
● ceftazidime
● co-amoxiclav
● diazepam emulsion
● dopexamine
● doxorubicin
● etoposide
● hydrocortisone
● ranitidine
● salbutamol
● vancomycin

The calculations involved are not complex, but as with all calculations, accuracy is essential.

EXAMPLE 1

Dopexamine is to be diluted to produce a solution containing 400 micrograms in 1 mL. To prepare 100 mL of the dilute solution, the total amount of dopexamine required is:

100×400 micrograms = 40 000 micrograms

Convert to mg:

$$\frac{40000}{1000} = 40 \, mg$$

The solution available for dilution contains 10 mg in 1 mL in 5 mL ampoules (or 50 mg in 5 mL).

Applying the formula,

$$\frac{\text{Want}}{\text{Got}} \times \text{Volume} = \frac{40\text{mg}}{50\text{mg}} \times 5\text{mL}$$

$$= 4\text{mL}$$

4 mL must be diluted to 100 mL to provide a solution containing 400 micrograms in 1 mL.

EXAMPLE 2

Atosiban is to be diluted to a concentration of 750 micrograms/mL. Prepare 100 mL of dilute solution for IV infusion.

Amount of atosiban required is

100 × 750 micrograms = 75 000 micrograms

Convert to mg:

$$\frac{75000}{1000} = 75\text{mg}$$

The solution available for dilution contains 7.5 mg in 1 mL in 5 mL vials.

Applying the formula,

$$\frac{\text{Want}}{\text{Got}} \times \text{Volume} = \frac{75\text{mg}}{7.5\text{mg}} \times 1\text{mL}$$

$$= 10\text{mL}$$

10 mL is diluted to 100 mL.

EXAMPLE 3

Salbutamol solution for infusion should contain 200 micrograms in 1 mL. To prepare 200 mL of the dilute solution, the total amount of salbutamol required is

200 × 200 micrograms = 40 000 micrograms

Convert to mg:

$$\frac{40000}{1000} = 40\text{mg}$$

The solution available for dilution contains 1 mg/1 mL in 5 mL ampoules (or 5 mg in 5 mL).

Applying the formula,

$$\frac{\text{Want}}{\text{Got}} \times \text{Volume} = \frac{40\,\text{mg}}{5\,\text{mg}} \times 5\,\text{mL}$$
$$= 40\,\text{mL}$$

Transfusion of blood and blood components

It is essential when administering blood or its components to use the correct administration set, normally one that delivers 15 drops/minute.

The volume in each bag (referred to by staff as a unit and by the patient as a pint) of blood varies to an extent and so it is important to read the accompanying blood prescription form to establish the exact volume.

For example, a bag of red cells may contain anything from 260 mL to 300 mL. The figure could be 268 mL. If the bag is to be transfused in 3 hours, to calculate the flow rate, the volume, as before, must be divided by the duration:

$$\frac{268\,\text{mL}}{3\,\text{h}} = \frac{268\,\text{mL}}{180\,\text{min}}$$
$$= 1.489\,\text{mL}$$

To calculate the number of drops per minute, 1.489 is multiplied by 15 (remember, the administration set used for blood transfusion is set at 15 drops per mL):

Number of drops/min = 22.33 (rounded down = 22)

An example such as this one should be checked using a calculator.

Subcutaneous infusion

A number of medicines can be infused into the body by the subcutaneous route; the administration of a subcutaneous infusion can be established and maintained by the nurse. The introduction of fluid into the patient by this method is dependent on gravity; there is no need for an infusion pump to be used. Alternatively, a syringe driver may be used.

Clear fluids are always used and so the administration set is always the same, i.e. one that is set at 20 drops per mL. Calculating the flow rate is exactly the same as for a gravity-assisted intravenous infusion (see p. 126).

Large volume parenteral calculations

The calculations in this section are presented in a different format. Because the prescribing documentation and calculations are very varied, the classification system used earlier is not appropriate. All the essential information is given to enable the calculations to be completed using the methods covered in the text. Answers are given on p. 150.

Exercise 5.27

Prescription/other clinical data

Foscarnet 60 mg/kg every 8 hours via central IV line

Product details

Foscarnet sodium hexahydrate 24 mg in 1 mL (250 mL container)

Commentary

Patient's weight is 15 kg

Calculations

(a) What is the dose (mg) to be given every 8 hours?
(b) What is the volume (mL) containing the required dose?

Exercise 5.28

Prescription/other clinical data

Human actrapid (soluble human insulin) 50 units in 50 mL 0.9% sodium chloride solution (for use in syringe driver)

Product details

Human actrapid insulin 100 units/1 mL

Calculations

(a) What is the volume (mL) of insulin injection to be made up to 50 mL?
(b) What is the volume of sodium chloride solution (mL) to be used?

Exercise 5.29

Prescription/other clinical data

Dopamine 260 mg IV to be diluted to 1.6 mg/1 mL

Product details

Dopamine injection 50 mg/1 mL (in 5 mL ampoules)

Calculations

(a) What is the volume (mL) of dopamine injection required?
(b) What is the *total* volume (mL) of the solution to be given?

Exercise 5.30

Prescription/other clinical data

Sodium bicarbonate 50 mmol by IV injection

Product details

Sodium bicarbonate 1.26% w/v sterile solution containing 150 mmol each of Na$^+$ and HCO$_3^-$ per litre

Calculation

What is the total volume (mL) of sodium bicarbonate solution to be infused?

Exercise 5.31

Prescription/other clinical data

Digoxin 500 micrograms IV to be given over a 2 hour period diluted in 50 mL glucose 5% solution

Product details

Digoxin injection 250 micrograms/1 mL in 2 mL ampoules

Calculations

(a) What is the volume (mL) of the digoxin injection?
(b) How much diluent (mL) is required?

Exercise 5.32

Prescription/other clinical data

Aminophylline 1 mg/kg/hour by IV infusion

Commentary

Patient's weight is 30 kg

Product details

Aminophylline 250 mg in 500 mL sodium chloride solution 0.9%

Calculations

(a) Calculate the quantity (mg) of aminophylline to be given each hour
(b) Calculate the flow rate in mL/hour

Exercise 5.33

Prescription/other clinical data

Lidocaine 1 mg/minute by IV infusion

Product details

Lidocaine 1 g in 500 mL glucose 5% w/v solution

Calculation

Calculate the flow rate in mL/hour

Exercise 5.34

Prescription/other clinical data

Vasopressin 0.2 unit/1 mL to be given over 15 minutes IV

Product details

Synthetic vasopressin injection 20 units/1 mL in 1 mL ampoules

Commentary

Diluent to be used: 5% w/v glucose solution (100 mL)

Calculation

Calculate the volume of vasopressin injection (mL) to be diluted to 100 mL

Exercise 5.35

Prescription/other clinical data

Heparin 500 units/1 mL in 50 mL glucose solution 5% by continuous IV infusion

Product details

Heparin injection 25 000 units/1 mL in 1 mL ampoules

Calculation

Calculate the total quantity (mL) of heparin injection to be diluted to 50 mL

Exercise 5.36

Prescription/other clinical data

Adrenaline (epinephrine) 50 mL of a 1 in 10 000 solution infused IV at 5 mL/hour

Product details

Adrenaline 1 in 10 000 injection

Calculation

How much adrenaline (micrograms) is infused per hour?

Examples 5.37–5.40 are not based on prescriptions but are included as an aid to understanding percentages.

Exercise 5.37

Product details

Sodium chloride 0.18% w/v and glucose 4% w/v in 500 mL bag

Calculations

(a) Calculate the quantity of sodium chloride (mg) in 500 mL
(b) Calculate the quantity of glucose (g) in 500 mL

Exercise 5.38

Product details

Sodium bicarbonate 8.4% w/v

Calculation

What is the concentration of sodium bicarbonate in the solution (mg/mL)?

Exercise 5.39

Product details

Sodium bicarbonate 1.26% w/v (relative molecular weight of sodium bicarbonate is 84 g)

Calculations

(a) Calculate the concentration of sodium bicarbonate in mmol per litre
(b) Calculate the concentration of sodium bicarbonate in mmol/mL

Exercise 5.40

Product details

Glucose 5% w/v solution

Calculations

(a) Calculate the quantity (g) of glucose in 1 litre solution
(b) Calculate the quantity of glucose (g) in 50 mL solution

REFERENCES

Reynard C, Kindlen M, Aport S 2004 Procedures in palliative care. Worksheet. Coleman Education Centre, St. Oswald's Hospice, Newcastle-upon-Tyne.

Abbreviations

BAN	British Approved Name
BMI	body mass index
BN	batch number
BNF	British National Formulary
BP	British Pharmacopoeia
BPC	British Pharmaceutical Codex
BSA	body surface area
cap.	capsule
CD	Controlled Drug
DV	displacement value
E-number	code number designating additives to a medicine according to EU directives
e/c	enteric-coated
EP	European Pharmacopoeia
Exp.	expiry date
g	gram
h	hour
IM	intramuscular
INR	international normalised ratio
IV	intravenous
IVI	intravenous infusion
kg	kilogram
L	litre (L is rarely used)
mg	milligram
mL (ml)	millilitre
mmol	millimole

m/r	modified-release
mol	mole
P	pharmacy medicine
Ph. Eur.	European Pharmacopoeia
PL	product licence
POM	prescription-only medicine
®	registered trademark
rINN	Recommended International Non-proprietary Name
SC	subcutaneous
SI units	Système International (d'Unités)
tab.	tablet
™	trademark
*	trademark

APPENDIX B
Arithmetical signs

+	plus
−	minus
±	plus or minus
×	multiplied by ('times')
÷	divided by
=	equals
≡	equivalent to; identical with
≈	approximately equals
≃	approximately
<	less than
>	greater than
%	percent
∴	therefore
:	ratio of
/	ratio of

APPENDIX C

Glossary

Base. A chemical compound with alkaline properties

British Pharmaceutical Codex. Quality standard

British Pharmacopoeia. Quality standard

Calculation. The working out of a problem mathematically

Calculator. An electronic device that performs arithmetical calculations

Cancelling down. Dividing the numerator and denominator of a vulgar fraction by the same number

Centimetre. One hundredth of a metre

Compound preparation. A medicine containing more than one drug

Decimal. Numbered by tens

Decimal fraction. A fraction expressed using decimal notation, e.g. 0.5

Denominator. The lower number in a vulgar fraction

Digit. Any one of the Arabic numerals from 0 to 9

Diluent. A liquid used to reconstitute a powder to make a solution for oral or parenteral use, or a liquid used to produce a solution of lower concentration than the original solution

Dilution. A weaker preparation made by adding a calculated amount of a diluent to a more concentrated preparation

Displacement value. The volume of a diluent displaced by a powder or the increase in volume of a diluent caused by a solute

Dose/dosage. The amount of a drug expressed in metric units needed to produce a therapeutic response

Dyscalculia. Number dyslexia

Equation. A statement of the equality of two quantities, e.g. 14 + 9 = 23

Ester. A clinical compound of an alcohol with an acid

Even numbers. Every second number starting with the number 2 (e.g. 2, 4, 6, 8)

Excipient. A pharmacologically inactive substance included in a medicine in order to produce a convenient, stable and where appropriate palatable preparation

Fraction. A part of a whole

Gram. One-thousandth of a kilogram

Imperial measure. Non-metric measure or weight (e.g. pint, yard, pound)

Ion. Atom or molecule that has acquired an electrical charge by the loss or gain of one or more electrons

Kilogram. One thousand grams

Label. The quantitative and qualitative information conveyed on the package of a medicine

Length. Extent from end to end

Litre. One thousand millilitres

Microgram. One-thousandth of a milligram

Milligram. One-thousandth of a gram

Millimetre. One-thousandth of a metre

Mole. One mole of a drug weighs (in grams) the same as the relative molecular mass of that drug

Nanogram. One-thousandth of a microgram

Nomogram. A graphical presentation used to determine body surface area from height and mass

Numeracy. The ability to solve arithmetical problems

Numerals. *Arabic:* numerals normally used in arithmetic, written as 1, 2, 3, etc. *Roman:* numerals written as letters, e.g. III, VII, XI

Numerator. Upper number of a vulgar fraction

Odd numbers. Every second number, starting with the number 1 (e.g. 1, 3, 5, 7)

Overage. The amount of solution present in an ampoule in excess of the nominal volume in the ampoule, which enables the correct volume to be measured

Percentage. Parts per 100; value expressed in hundredths

Picogram. One-thousandth of a nanogram

Proportion. The relation of one thing to another in magnitude

Proprietary name. Brand or trade name

Reconstitution. Restoring the constitution of a dried medicine by adding liquid

Salt. A chemical compound formed by reacting an acid plus base

Simplifying. Reducing an arithmetical configuration, such as a fraction, to its simplest form

Solute. A substance dissolved in a liquid (solvent) to produce a solution

Units of activity. An expression used to indicate the strength of some medicines

Volume. Quantity of liquid

Vulgar fraction. A portion of a quantity written with one number above another separated by a line, e.g. $\frac{3}{4}$

Weight (mass). Quantity determined by weighing

Whole number. Any number that is not a fraction and does not have a fraction added to it

APPENDIX D

Self-assessment

Twenty questions now follow. Most of the information needed to address them is contained within the text.

Answers may be found on pp. 151–152

1. What is meant by 'SI units'?

2. What does POM stand for?

3. Express the following abbreviations in full:
   (a) w/w
   (b) v/v
   (c) w/v
   (d) v/w

4. What should you do if the answer to a drug calculation is not what you expect it to be?

5. Name the main sources of drug information available to the nurse.

6. What does the expression 1 in 1000 mean?

7. Why should you never split or break a coated or slow-release tablet before administration?

8. What is meant by a meniscus?

9. Why might a label in the UK contain information other than in English?

10. Complete the following:

    kilogram
    gram

    microgram

    picogram

11. How many micrograms are there in one milligram?
    (a) 10
    (b) 100
    (c) 1000
    (d) 10000

12. The following components *must* appear on a medicine label. One is missing. What is it?

Pharmacy address
No. of dosage units dispensed
Expiry date
Warning
Batch no.
Approved name of drug
Formulation

13. Match the following with the quantities in the boxes:
    (a) 1000 mg
    (b) 1500 mg
    (c) 250 micrograms
    (d) 500 mg

(1) 1.5 g	
(2) 0.25 mg	
(3) 0.5 g	
(4) 1 g	

14. Name two drugs where the dose is expressed in units.

15. Why is a calculation not normally needed when administering a compound preparation, e.g. co-prenocide?

16. Why are approved names preferred to proprietary names?

17. Complete the following:

Decimal	Fraction	Percentage
0.75	$\frac{3}{4}$	75%
		10%
0.6		
	$\frac{1}{4}$	
	$\frac{1}{2}$	
0.2		
		5%

18. Express 1.2 g in milligrams.

19. Express one litre in millilitres.

20. What does the word parenteral mean?

APPENDIX **E**

Answers to questions about labels (Chapter 1)

Label 1.1

1. Doxepin
2. No. It would be issued on prescription only
3. Yes
4. 2

Label 1.2

1. The strength of the eye drops; 0.3 g of active ingredient in 100 mL of the product (i.e. weight in volume)
2. 10 mL
3. Discard 28 days after opening
4. The product may be bought over the counter in a pharmacy

Label 1.3

1. Trade mark
2. Coating on a tablet which remains intact in the acid conditions of the stomach but dissolves in the higher pH of the intestine
3. The brand or trade name
4. The European Pharmacopoeia
5. Do not take indigestion remedies at the same time of day as this medicine
   Steroid card
   Swallow whole; do not chew

Label 1.4

1. Registered trade mark
2. No. It contains egg phospholipids
3. Product licence
4. Intravenous

APPENDIX F
Answers to calculations

Chapter 2

Page 17
(a) 0.75
(b) 1.5
(c) 0.25
(d) 0.1
(e) 0.4

Page 18
(a) $\frac{1}{10}$
(b) $\frac{1}{2}$
(c) $\frac{1}{4}$
(d) $\frac{3}{4}$
(e) $\frac{1}{5}$

Chapter 4

Level I

4.1   2 tablets

4.2   4 capsules

4.3   2 tablets

4.4 $1\frac{1}{2}$ tablets

4.5 $1\frac{1}{2}$ tablets

4.6 $\frac{1}{2}$ a tablet

4.7   12 tablets

4.8   One 5 mg tablet and one 1 mg tablet (*or* two 3 mg tablets)

4.9   3 capsules

4.10 2 tablets

4.11 4 tablets

4.12 $\frac{1}{2}$ a tablet

4.13 3 tablets

4.14 2 tablets

4.15 2 tablets

4.16 2 tablets

4.17 2 tablets

4.18 3 tablets

4.19 $1\frac{1}{2}$ tablets

Level II

4.20 20 mL syrup

4.21 2.5 mL suspension

4.22 ½ a tablet

4.23 2 tablets

4.24 7.5 mL oral solution

4.25 2 capsules

4.26 1 tablet

4.27 10 mL suspension

4.28 2 tablets

4.29 7.5 mL suspension

4.30 6 mL syrup

4.31 2 inhalations

4.32 20 mL syrup

4.33 10 mL liquid

4.34 15 mL syrup

4.35 15 mL elixir

4.36 0.75 mL oral solution

4.37 15 mL suspension

4.38 1 tablet

4.39 16 mL oral solution

4.40 2.5 mL oral solution

4.41 7.5 mL oral suspension

4.42 3 tablets

4.43 10 mL suspension

4.44 2.5 mL suspension

Level III

4.45 2 tablets

4.46 1.25 mL solution

4.47 2.5 mL nebuliser solution

4.48 30 mL syrup

4.49 0.7 mL suspension

4.50 0.2 mL oral solution

4.51 1.5 mL elixir

4.52 1.5 mL oral solution

4.53 1 mL oral solution

4.54 6.25 mL oral suspension

4.55 2.5 mL oral solution

4.56 1 tablet three times a day

4.57 4 tablets

4.58 4 capsules

4.59 2 tablets

4.60 $\frac{1}{2}$ a tablet

4.61 20 mL suspension

4.62 2 tablets

4.63 1.5 mL suspension

4.64 15 mL suspension

4.65 20 mL suspension

4.66 4 mL elixir

Chapter 5

SMALL VOLUME

Level I

5.1   0.25 mL IM injection

5.2   0.25 mL IV injection

5.3   1 mL IM injection

5.4   0.2 mL IV injection

Level II

5.5   1.5 mL IM injection

5.6   0.666 rep. mL (give 0.7 mL in adult; seek advice for child) IM injection

5.7   1.5 mL IV injection

5.8   1.5 mL IV injection

5.9   0.4 mL SC injection

5.10 0.25 mL IV injection

5.11 0.75 mL IV injection

5.12 0.6 mL IV injection

5.13 0.2 mL IV injection; 0.8 mL IV injection

Level III

5.14 0.2 mL SC injection

5.15 0.25 mL IM injection

5.16 0.4 mL IM injection

5.17 6 mL IV injection

5.18 0.5 mL IM injection

5.19 4 mL IV injection; 20 mL IV injection

5.20 4 mL IM injection

5.21 0.02 mL IV injection

5.22 0.75 mL SC injection

5.23 0.5 mL IM injection

5.24 0.25 mL intra-articular injection

5.25 0.5 mL slow IV injection

5.26 4 mL IM injection

LARGE VOLUME

5.27 (a) 900 mg; (b) 37.5 mL

5.28 (a) 0.5 mL; (b) 49.5 mL

5.29 (a) 5.2 mL; (b) 162.5 mL

5.30 333 mL

5.31 (a) 2 mL; (b) 48 mL

5.32 (a) 30 mg; (b) 60 mL

5.33 30 mL

5.34 1 mL

5.35 1 mL

5.36 500 micrograms

5.37 (a) 900 mg; (b) 20 g

5.38 84 mg

5.39 (a) 150 mmol/litre; (b) 0.15 mmol/mL

5.40 (a) 50 g; (b) 2.5 g

Answers to self-assessment

1. Universal system of weights and measures which is used to express the strength of a medicine – the metric system

2. Prescription-only medicine

3. (a) Weight in weight
   (b) Volume in volume
   (c) Weight in volume
   (d) Volume in weight

4. Do not administer the medicine;
   check your calculation again;
   try using another method;
   ask a reliable colleague to make an independent calculation;
   refer back to the prescriber

5. British National Formulary (BNF)
   Product literature or Data Sheet Compendium
   Local medicine information service

6. 1 g in 1000 mL or 1 mg in 1 mL

7. It could destroy the properties of the tablet and cause irritation or premature release of the drug into an incompatible pH in the gastrointestinal tract

8. The curve formed at the surface of a liquid in a container

9. It may be more economical for health authorities/retail outlets to purchase a product from overseas (parallel imports)

10. Milligram; nanogram

11. (c) 1000

12. Strength of the product

13. (1) and (b); (2) and (c); (3) and (d); (4) and (a)

14. Heparin, insulin

15. They are unique preparations with fixed proportion of ingredients, prescribed as numbers of tablets or volume of liquid

16. They are safer to use since they are universally recognised

17.

Decimal	Fraction	Percentage
0.1	$\frac{1}{10}$	10%
0.6	$\frac{3}{5}$	60%
0.25	$\frac{1}{4}$	25%
0.5	$\frac{1}{2}$	50%
0.2	$\frac{1}{5}$	20%
0.05	$\frac{1}{20}$	5%

18. 1200 mg

19. 1000 mL

20. Other than the alimentary canal; by injection

Index